T0007243

The Treadwell's Book
of Plant Magic

The Treadwell's Book of Plant Magic

Christina Oakley Harrington

WEISER BOOKS

This edition first published in 2023 by Weiser Books, an imprint of

Red Wheel/Weiser, LLC
With offices at:
65 Parker Street, Suite 7
Newburyport, MA 01950
www.redwheelweiser.com

Copyright © 2023 by Christina Oakley Harrington
All rights reserved. No part of this publication may be reproduced or transmitted
in any form or by any means, electronic or mechanical, including photocopying,
recording, or by any information storage and retrieval system, without permission in writing from Red Wheel/Weiser, LLC. Reviewers may quote brief passages.
Previously published in 2020 by Treadwell's Books.

ISBN: 978-1-57863-801-7
Library of Congress Cataloging-in-Publication Data available on request.

Cover design by Tom Etherington
Interior by Twisted Trunk
Typeset in ITC Garamond

Printed in the United States of America
IBI
10   9   8   7   6   5   4   3   2   1

This book contains advice and information for using herbs and other botanicals, and is not meant to diagnose, treat, or prescribe. It should be used to supplement, not replace, the advice of your physician or other trained healthcare practitioner. If you know or suspect you have a medical condition, are experiencing physical symptoms, or if you feel unwell, seek your physician's advice before embarking on any medical program or treatment. Readers are cautioned to follow instructions carefully and accurately for the best effect. Readers using the information in this book do so entirely at their own risk, and the author and publisher accept no liability if adverse effects are caused.

Introduction and Acknowledgements

This guide is for explorers of herb magic—people who wish to use plants, twigs, flowers and fruit in their practice. The uses presented here all come from folk tradition, and their efficacy has been attested over hundreds of years. So often, the powers of the plant spirits are forgotten, and I hope in this book to bring them back to wider appreciation and recognition.

As Britain and Europe were overtaken with rationalism and superstitions died away in the nineteenth century, so too did the old knowledge of these plant usages; as people are once again drawn to herbal magics, they are often frustrated in finding knowledge about the herbs in their local eco-systems. As a result, there has been a surge of use of plants from other continents, in uses that are both ecologically exploitative and unwittingly culturally appropriative. Two of the most visible cases are white sage from North America and Palo Santo from South America. This book greets native practitioners from around the world with fraternal respect, though I urge readers to forage locally; the European plants in this book are powerful, useful and effective. We bring them to the cauldron, and to the altar. All who read this book I warmly invite to explore these plants, to get to know them, talk to them and ask their help in the ways our forebears did for so many centuries.

Many thanks are in order at the opening of this book. It could not have been written without the work and support of many people. I must first acknowledge my colleagues at Treadwell's; their professionalism, warmth and competence never cease to amaze me, and it is because of their support that I have had the time to complete this book. I thank also my family. And I extend my gratitude to those who are my fellow travellers in the old ways, especially those in my closest circle.

The dedication, though, is to the one who shares my life and my heart. Becky, this is for you.

February 2020

Problems and Solutions

To find which herb you need, find your current concern on the list below, then turn to the entry which discusses the listed plant or tree. If more than one herb is suitable, look for plants which are handily available to you. If you have a choice among those, you're very lucky indeed; in that case, read closely through the entries on the relevant herbs, then choose the one (or ones) which seem the most appropriate.

Abundance – apple; *see also* money, if it is financial
   abundance you seek

Admittance, gaining – *see* doors

Anger, dispelling – fig
   restraint from actions taken in anger – rue

Animal wellbeing – ash
   communication – clubmoss
   return home – holly
   protection from attack – herb bennet

Anxiety – betony, borage, thistle; see also mental and
   psychological distress, countering

Athletics, speed – motherwort, mugwort
   endurance – St John's wort

Attractiveness – lady's mantle, marigold, saxifrage, valerian

Authority, to gain – oak
   for women – rosemary, sage

Baby blessing – ash, birch, butterwort, cloves, hawthorn,
   peony, vervain, yarrow

1

Problems and Solutions

Bee blessing – balm

Bereavement – *see* death

Betrayal – poplar

Breaking contracts – poplar

Bulletproofing – amaranth, fuller's teasel, pine

Caves – *see* underground

Child blessing – daisy, mistletoe, rose, vervain

Conflict, creating – *see* discord

Coronation – 'Coronation Oil'

Courage – borage, catnip, thyme

Curse, undoing – box, walnut; *see also* 'Tyrolian
    Unbewitching Spell'

Death, as a theme – cypress, pine

    blessing the dead – juniper

    grief – willow

    remembrance – rosemary

Desirability – marigold, valerian

Desire – *see* passion

Bad people, detecting – chamomile, clover, ground ivy, ivy,
    saxifrage, walnut, 'Tyrolian Witch Viewer' spell

Difficult conversations – vervain

Discord, creating – bay, catnip, 'To Create Disharmony' spell

    ending – mint, valerian, vervain

Doctors – peony

Doors, opening locked – caper spurge, chicory, honesty,
    mistletoe, sesame, savory, vervain

Dragons, encountering – lime tree

Dreams, peaceful – *see* nightmares

prophetic – bay, chasteberry, elder, poppy, rosemary, vervain,
    'St Agnes's Prophetic Dream Spell', 'St Luke's Prophecy
    Spell'

Enemies, making peace among – mint, valerian

    creating – bay, catnip

Evil eye, protection against – angelica, beech, birch, bog
    myrtle, garlic, holly, hyssop, juniper, periwinkle,
    rowan, rue, wormwood

Exam success – mint

Exorcism – 'Exorcism Water'

Fairies, encountering – alder, cinquefoil, clover, cowslip,
    elder, fern, fig, forget-me-not, greater stitchwort,
    hawthorn, herb robert, lime tree, oak, primrose,
    rowan, saxifrage, self-heal, thyme, walnut, willow,
    rowan, 'To See Fairies' spell

    granting wishes – oak

    answering questions – 'To Call the Fairy Sisters' spell

Faithfulness, enforcing – caraway, clover, parsley

Fame and honour – bay

Favour, gaining through networking – valerian

Favours, gaining from tree spirits: elder, fir, oak

    getting someone to grant you – cinquefoil

Female gender – fig, ivy, sage

Financial success – *see* wealth

Finding lost objects – *see* lost object, finding

Folly, restraining actions of – rue

Friendship, attracting – marigold, rosemary

    cementing – basil

    filling the home – lime tree, mistletoe, vervain

    rekindling – yarrow

Future, ability to see – Prophecy Perfume; *see also* dreams

Gambling luck – clover, St John's blood

Ghosts, seeing – mistletoe

Gossip, stopping – Against Slander spell

Good luck, good fortune – apple wood (Yule), ash, clover,
    hawthorn (May Day), oak, rowan, thyme, wormwood
    (midsummer)

Happiness – balm, borage, crocus (saffron)

Heartbreak, healing – balm, borage, pansy, willow

Problems and Solutions

Home blessing – lime tree, mistletoe, myrtle, St John's wort

Influence, gaining – valerian

Insomnia – *see* sleep, causing profound

Invincibility – *see* bulletproofing

Invisibility – amaranth, fern, hazel

Jealousy and envy, protecting against – dill; *see also* evil eye; this is the term used for the perceived dangerous energy created by a person's ill-wishing jealousy

Joy – crocus (saffron)

Justice, obtaining – lime tree

Liars, detecting – clover

Lost object, finding – juniper, yew

Love, making it subside – amaranth

   blessings for couples – bay, birch, lime tree, marigold, marjoram, vervain

   making a lover return – bay, daisy

   with passion, arousing – crocus (saffron)

   attracting a lover – love-in-a-mist, marigold, pansy, poppy, purslane, rose, valerian

   attracting a dreamy love – poppy

   drawing love very quickly – ash, basil, pansy

   rekindling – dill, periwinkle; 'Rekindling Love' spell

   making a chosen person love you – basil, cyclamen, sage, valerian, vervain

   resisting love spells put upon you – alder

   showing and strengthening – birch

   ending a relationship – willow

   passionate – *see* passion and sex

   lovesickness – *see* heartbreak

Loyalty – *see* faithfulness

Luck – ash; see also gambling luck

Magic, becoming adept – crocus (saffron), fern, periwinkle, vervain, 'To Believe Yourself a Witch' spell

Marriage, happy – *see* love

    manifesting – rose

Medical professionals – peony

Melancholy, countering – balm, betony, borage, hyssop, feverfew, milk thistle, St John's wort

    (uncommunicative), countering – feverfew

Male gender, representing – mandrake, pine

Membership – gaining entry to organisations with selective admission policies; *see* doors

Mental and psychological distress, countering – agrimony, balm, bay, betony, borage, daffodil, feverfew, herb paris, honesty, periwinkle, rue, thistle, thyme, vervain

Military service, to evade – clover

Mining – pomegranate, primrose, sesame

Money, wealth – marigold, vervain

Negotiation, achieving amicable and successful – vervain

Nightmares, curing – fir, mistletoe, periwinkle, rosemary

Oathbreaking – poplar

Passion, arousing – dill

    arousing it quickly – basil

    calming and fading – amaranth, chasteberry

    restraining acts of – rue

    reviving in a partner – dill, periwinkle; see also 'Rekindling Love' spell

Patrons and patronage, gaining – chicory

Peace truce, effecting – mint, valerian, vervain

Persuasion, succeeding in – cinquefoil

Pets – *see* animal wellbeing

Poppets, human image magic – fig, holly, ivy, mandrake, white bryony

Popularity, gaining – marigold

Power over another person – cypress, lime tree

Prayers, achieving answers – beech

Problems and Solutions

Protection against curses – garlic

    at sea – hazel, pine

    around death – cypress

    from bad people – marjoram, peony, pomegranate, poplar

    from jealousy and envy; see evil eye, protection against

    from physical attack, herb bennet, purslane

    during travel – wormwood

    against travel theft – vervain, wormwood

    against theft at home – fir

    from a stalker, unwanted admirer or ex-lover – willow

Protection of your person – agrimony, alder (with care), angelica, aniseed, ash, bay, beech, bog myrtle, box, butterwort, chervil, cloves, clubmoss, hazel, holly, juniper, marjoram, mugwort, parsley, pimpernel, rose, rowan, St John's blood, St John's wort, thyme, vervain, walnut, woodruff, yarrow, yew

Protection of home or other space – agrimony, angelica, bay, birch, caper spurge, chamomile, cyclamen, elder (midsummer only), fennel, hawthorn, herb bennet, holly, hyssop, juniper, parsley, primrose, rosemary, rowan, thyme, vervain, woodruff, yarrow, yew

    of city homes and spaces – olive, St John's wort

Resilience – chamomile

Restraint – rue

Revenge – *see* betrayal

Risks and entrepreneurship – clover, St John's blood

Running success – motherwort, mugwort, St John's wort

Sailing, seafaring protection – hazel, pine

Secrets, keeping – rose

Sex, having good – mugwort, myrtle

    drawing sex – crocus (saffron), pine, pansy, savory

becoming sexually appealing – valerian

obsession, calming – amaranth, chasteberry

Shooting, hitting targets – St John's blood, 'To Hit a Target' spell

Sleep, causing profound – agrimony

Sponsorship, gaining – chicory

Strength – ash, crocus (saffron), elder, oak, woodruff

Subways, metros, magic in – pomegranate, primrose, sesame

Success in a large project – aniseed

Theft, prevention during travel – vervain, wormwood

to catch a thief – 'To Catch a Thief' spell

return of stolen items – juniper

Tools, magical – birch, broom, elder, hazel, purslane

Travel, energy during – mugwort, St John's wort

preventing theft during – wormwood, vervain

safety – clover

Treasure, finding – cowslips, fern

Underground endeavours – pomegranate, primrose, sesame

Wealth – marigold, vervain

Wisdom, gaining – hazel

Worry, calming – balm, thistle, 'Disastrous Imaginings' spell

Agnus Castus
See chasteberry

Agrimony
Also known as stickwort or sticklewort
Genus *Agrimonia*. Attribution: Jupiter (Culpeper)
Agrimony is one of the more important magical herbs of the British Isles. It is a spiky wildflower whose little yellow five-petalled flowers cling to the tall stem. It grows plentifully in England and Wales, more rarely in Scotland. In both Scotland and England it has been recognised as a plant of protection as far back as the early Middle Ages.[1] It is known by many local names and has been used for good purposes throughout the centuries. A seventeenth-century London cunning man's book prescribes that, 'if any be in danger of witchcraft let them carry about them ... stickwort, and they will be free of it'.[2] In a Scottish witch trial in the eighteenth century, agrimony is cited as being a witch cure for elf-shot, a mysterious illness attributed to attack by supernatural beings.[3] Its powers against evil forces were known in Germany, too. Hildegard of Bingen, the medieval medical expert, used agrimony in a treatment for mental illness.

> Let a person who has lost understanding and knowledge have the hair cut from his or her head since the hair creates a horrible shaking tremor. Then cook agrimony in water and wash the person's head with this warm water. Also, the herb should be tied warm over the heart when the person first senses mindlessness. Then place it warm over the forehead and temples. The person's understanding and knowledge will be purified, and the mindlessness will leave.

The use of agrimony in treating mental distress has a long history, as we see from a fifteenth-century charm: to cure delusion and insanity, it was advised that you tie a sprig of agrimony to your arm; if you do so, you will be returned to your right state of mind—if you are a man, tie it to your right arm; if you are a woman, put it on the left.[4]

Agrimony also has the magical power to put a person to sleep and keep them unconscious; one old British source says that if you place a sprig of common agrimony under a person's pillow, they will sleep until it is removed. This power is expressed in the old English rhyme, here modernised:

> If it be laid under a man's head,
> He shall sleep as if he were dead;
> He shall never dread nor waken
> Till from under his head it be taken.[5]

Agrimony is thus a wonderful plant to use in spells to counter insomnia and nightmares.

∞　**Agrimony for sleep.** If you are fortunate enough to have agrimony growing near you, it is good to pluck it fresh, first addressing the plant and asking it for its help. You can of course used dried agrimony, which can be bought online. We suggest that you prepare your agrimony on a Thursday, the day of Jupiter (the ruler of its powers) or on a Monday, the day of the moon and thus of sleep. The simplest way of using it for sleep is to put a little under your pillow, ideally in a piece of blue, white or purple fabric tied in a ribbon of one of those colours. A nice touch is to put a small bit of silver metal in the wrap, to enhance the lunar sleep energies, perhaps a silver earring or pendant.

∞　Alternatively, on a Monday, fill the bathroom or kitchen sink with agrimony herbal 'tea' (place a handful of the herb into the sink and pour boiling water over it). Then add some more warm water and a small item of silver; again, an earring will do. Place your pillowcase in the sink and let the herbal mixture infuse into the fabric. After you have soaked it for some time, dry the pillowcase, then place it back on your pillow, with the piece of silver underneath.

∞　**Agrimony for protection.** As it brings blessing, wellness and protection from ill fortune, agrimony is good to place around yourself and wherever you spend the most time. It is a pretty wildflower which goes well in summer bouquets; if you live in England or Wales, there is probably some growing in your neighbourhood. If you don't have any locally and are using dried agrimony, you can make agrimony herbal tea, a traditional spring drink in parts of France. If you want to make a ceremony of your tea drinking, do it on a Thursday and use a purple cup and wear some purple clothing. Another option is to make a protection/blessing packet. On a small square of paper or card, draw the symbol of Jupiter, place a pinch of dried agrimony in the middle then fold and seal the card with wax or string, ideally purple. Carry this little wrap around with you in your daily life.

∞ **Agrimony in magic against psychic disequilibrium.** As the uses mentioned above show, agrimony is a herb that has long been used in magical spells for people who are unsettled and/or suffering from mental illness. We would stress that it is not a medical treatment, nor even a herbal remedy; we urge people to seek medical and psychological treatments from trained professionals and to follow their guidance faithfully. The agrimony spells may help the person to find the right doctor, to have the good fortune to be prescribed the correct medication, or to gain the clarity to undertake their practitioner's advice. Do your mental wellness spell on a Thursday. First speak to the agrimony plant and ask its help. Do this even if you are addressing chopped, dried agrimony you have bought. Make a large bowl of agrimony tea, about a gallon, then let it cool enough for you to rinse your head and hair with it. Alternatively, mix some agrimony with some oil (olive oil works well) in a pestle and mortar or blender, then, when you have a quiet hour, gently place this mixture on to your body, particularly in the heart region; also, affix some of it to your arms, left and right, with wide strips of fabric. We advise doing this in a warm room with low lighting and perhaps while playing soft music.

Alder

Alnus glutinosa. Attribution: Venus (Culpeper)
The alder is a tall-growing tree which is found near wetlands. Across Europe, the alder prompts wariness—possibly because it grows in deserted, marshy places and its wood, when cut,

11

is eerily red. In Somerset, it is considered a dangerous tree because unnamed supernatural beings—probably fairies—live in alder groves. If you go into a grove of alders, it is said you will never come back out because 'they will keep you'.[6] The Irish consider it bad luck to cut the alder down, presumably because it is home to supernatural beings.[7] Danish people assert that you can see the king of the fairies and his retinue if you stand under the alder at noon on Midsummer's Day.[8] Due to people's fear of the alder, it became a place of refuge for illicit lovers and outlaws.[9]

In Germany, there is a belief that alders have sentient consciousness: they say that the tree starts weeping when it hears people talk about cutting it down, even shedding drops of blood to beg for its life.[10] In spite of its reputation as a tree of ill fortune, however, people in some parts of Germany believe it has the power of protection against bad luck and bad magic.[11] Moreover, you can neutralise a love spell put upon you if you drink some alder-bark wine (add alder bark to wine and heat it).[12]

෨ **Alder for contacting fairies.** It is among the alders that you are very likely to succeed if you are making a pilgrimage to make contact with local spirits. First, find your nearest cluster of alders, looking initially near bodies of water in your area. Then, plan a long, unhurried walk to them and spend some time among them. A traditional day for such a project is Midsummer's Day, but if this is not convenient for you, we recommend doing it on the day or evening of the full moon. Bring an offering for the spirits: cream, milk or an alcoholic drink are known to be received favourably.

෨ **Alder for protection.** To use alder for blessing and protection, we recommend first spending some time with the tree and asking if it will give you its blessing. Proceed only if you are intuitively certain it gives you its good will; this is a tricksome tree and you would be wrong to assume it will be positively predisposed towards you. We recommend approaching trees and plants other than the alder for this reason; the exception would be if you had a strong and positive relationship with a particular alder tree.

∞   **Alder against others' love magic.** Drink alder-bark wine as outlined above.

Amaranth

Also known as love-lies-bleeding, prince's feather
Genus *Amaranthus*. Attribution: Saturn (Culpeper)
The ancient Greeks viewed the purple-flowered amaranth as a plant of eternal life, noting that its flowers do not fade or wilt after being plucked: in fact, the Greek word *amaranth* means 'not wilting'.[13] They believed that the fields of paradise were full of amaranth flowers. For this reason, it was used at funerals.[14]

Amaranth has specific magical powers, too. If you want to be invisible, wear a wreath of amaranth on Ascension Day.[15] Another of its powers is to curb affections; Nicholas Culpeper wrote that it is a plant of Saturn and thus 'an excellent qualifier of the unruly actions and passions of Venus, though Mars should also join with her'. Finally, in the early days of guns, amaranth was used to make a person bulletproof, as in this spell:

Amaranth Bulletproofing Spell

The first step is to find some *amaranthus hypochondriacus* [prince's feather] growing. Then, mark your diary for the next time a full moon falls on a Friday; this generally happens about once a year. When that night comes, go out at night under the full moon and find the plant. Pull up one plant of the amaranth by the roots. Take it home, clean the dirt off the roots, and then take the whole plant and prepare it so that you can wear it. This can be done by pressing it into a muslin bag or a small cotton pillowcase, then sew it into the lining of your jacket. If it is a small plant, you can put it into a small bag and wear it around your neck. Put this around your neck, or wear it some other way, when you are in danger of gunfire. Whoever wears it will not be hit by the shooter.[16]

∞   **Amaranth to calm passion.** Use amaranth in spells to make yourself or someone else fall out of love. It is useful in a spell to make two people lose their passion for one another, or to cause an unwanted admirer to lose interest in you. Such spells should be done on a Saturday, ideally during the waning moon, which is the two weeks after a full moon, when the moon appears smaller and smaller each night. The fortnight of the waning moon is the ideal time to do magic to make things wither, get smaller or go away.

∽ **Amaranth for invisibility.** There are any number of reasons a person may want to go about unnoticed but, whatever the reason, amaranth is a great help. The classic method is to make a wreath, using kitchen twist-ties or florist's wire, and wear it as a crown. The best day to make the crown and to do the invisibility spell is the dark of the moon, otherwise known as the new moon. On this day, the moon is herself invisible in the night sky. A quick look online will tell you when the new moon falls. If the new moon falls on a Saturday or a Wednesday (the night of trickster energy), you will be doubly lucky in the endeavour. A smaller bunch of amaranth tucked neatly into your hat, hood or pocket will also have the effect of making you succeed in escaping people's notice.

∽ **Amaranth in magic to become bulletproof.** A loving gift for a family member or friend who is going into a danger zone is to make them a charm bag including amaranth root, using the guidance given above. The most time-consuming part of the exercise may be finding where amaranth grows in your local area; alternatively, you may choose to buy a plant from a garden centre.

Angelica
Angelica archangelica. Attribution: Sun (Culpeper), Saturn (Lilly)
Angelica is a common wildflower with highly fragrant, light-coloured flowers which grow in bobble-like clumps on the stems. It has been an important herb for protection since Roman times: Fuchsius says wearing a bit of the root around your neck protects you from negative magic.[17] The name angelica comes from the dream of a monk in 1665 in which St Michael the Archangel appears and tells him to use it on plague victims.[18] Angelica is the only herb the herbalist Gerard cites as having power against witchcraft: he normally

14

avoids repeating superstitions. Much later English folklore says much the same, namely that you will be protected from the evil eye, or jealous evil magic, if you wear an angelica necklace.[19] Gypsies in Devon hang angelica over the door 'to ward off dark spirits'.[20]

∞ **Angelica for personal protection.** This is a herb we highly recommend for protection and blessing. If you are able to pluck it wild, please do so, making sure to first speak to the plant, attune to it and ask for its kindly goodwill. Only then should you uproot a plant or pluck it. The best day to prepare your spell is on a Sunday. Angelica is one of the herbs which is effective against the evil eye, namely the negative force which others' jealousy and hatred brings towards you. Mercifully, this is a rare misfortune, but when it does occur angelica is an excellent ally to call upon. For this we advise drying an angelica root, tying it with white ribbon or string then wearing it around your neck.

∞ **Angelica for house protection.** To keep your home full of light and clean energy, hang sprigs of angelica over your doorway. You may wish to put some over your windows as well. The angelica should have been picked, purchased or hung up on a Sunday, which is the day of light and wellbeing; it is itself a solar plant.

Aniseed

Pimpinella anisum. Attribution: Mercury (Culpeper, Lilly)[21] Aniseed has long been used in Europe to ward off evil.[22] As well as giving protection, aniseed also has the magical power to keep animals close to home; in Germany, aniseed oil was put in dovecotes to prevent the doves from flying away.[23] Aniseed is the key ingredient in the following success spell.

Old Aniseed Success Spell

This is a spell specifically 'if you are about to undertake any great task and wish to succeed in it'. Find somewhere, if possible, with an open fireplace. Set the fire, make an aniseed ointment [grind it with a small amount of oil in a mortar and pestle] and set it out with some red chalk and a pair of scissors. Start when it is late, well after dark, ideally about an hour before midnight, and make sure the fire is burning well. In silence, take the aniseed ointment and apply it to your head, then anoint your feet. Pick up the red chalk and draw a cross on your face and a large cross on your breast. Then take up the scissors and cut three locks of your hair from the back of your head. Set the hair down on the table and, standing in front of the fire, commit the three locks of hair to the flames, repeating the following verse without drawing a breath:

O sweet aniseed do assist me,
do assist in this, and I will bless thee;
For a great undertaking I want your aid,
Grant me the same and my fortune is made.

Watch the hair burn, then continue to watch the fire until the last spark has expired. Stay there until midnight, at which point go to bed, setting your alarm for 4 a.m. Rise and rinse off the aniseed ointment. Go to bed again, setting your alarm for 5 a.m. When the alarm goes off, get up and begin your work on the endeavour you wish to succeed in. If you do this spell correctly, you will have success in your great project.[24]

∞   **Aniseed for protection.** Keep some aniseed near you and around you to keep evil away.

∞   **Aniseed to stop pets from running away.** Pets running away is a worry for many owners. Aniseed is a useful magical aid in preventing a pet from or wandering off and getting lost. Place a bag of aniseed seeds (or a pot of aniseed oil) on a special shelf (or altar) next to a photograph of your pet, along with a bit of your pet's hair. Leave for a week, burning a green candle beside the photograph every night for a little while, say half an hour when it is quiet. Take some time to spend a special evening blessing your home as a place of return for your pet. Friday is the best day, during the full moon if possible. Go from room to room, spending time in each and filling it with a feeling of calm and bonding. Once you've done that, deposit a few seeds in each corner while continuing to have loving feelings about your animal. If you do not have seeds, a few drops of the oil will serve equally well. Conclude by doing this blessing to your front door, or your pet's favourite entrance to the home. Save the candle and the photograph in case your pet ever needs calling back home; if that happens, burn the candle again near the photo.

∞   **Aniseed for success.** Perform the Old Aniseed Success Spell above. You may need to modify it slightly for modern times.

Apple Tree
Malus domestica. Attribution: Venus (universal)
The Romans revered Pomona, goddess of fruit trees and fruit. Ever since then, the apple tree, above all others, has been seen as the tree of abundance, goodness and fertility. The apple is a benevolent spirit, revered especially in the west of England, where it is made into wassail in winter. The apple tree is chosen for the Yule log at Christmas, to bring good luck; sometimes, however, oak is chosen, for 'strength in the maister and safety from thunder'. The log must be burned on all of the twelve days of Christmas (25 December to 6 January).[25]

∞   **Apple wood for good luck.** Apple-tree wood has very potent powers to bring good fortune to a home. You need a fireplace, if you wish to do the traditional method of blessing your household. Search out apple-tree logs in your neighbourhood in December, gather or purchase plenty of them and give them attention: sprinklings of alcohol, offerings of scented oils (we like cinnamon oil), even songs. On the first of the twelve days of Christmas, start to put the logs on the fire, ideally one a day, with all the household gathered. Ask that they bring you good luck through the coming year.

∞   **Apples for creating abundance.** When you are looking to do magic for rich, sweet abundance, the apple is a wonderful fruit to use. If you are fortunate enough to live near an apple tree, using fruits from it will be best of all, as you will be drawing on the forces of the land where you live and with whom you share a local ecology. We personally enjoy apple spells around the act of baking them. An old-fashioned apple crumble or apple pie can be made ceremoniously of an evening in a candle-lit kitchen with harmonious music as an accompaniment. The best day is Friday, the day of abundance and love. Place a small token representing the thing you wish to flourish—a ring, a charm, or similar—into the pie before baking it. For any kind of abundance spell involving fruit, food or plants, ensure your portions are large—the spell is for largesse, so making large portions is part of the sympathetic magic.

Artemisia
See mugwort

Ash
Genus *fraxinus*. Common ash is *fraxinus excelsior*. Attribution: Sun (Culpeper, Lilly)
The ash is a very powerful tree with a long history of magical lore and use. Its mythic history is also rich. For the early Germanics, the ash is the world-tree under which all humanity lives and in whose upper leaves the gods dwell. In parts of Europe (Swabia, Tyrol), it is believed that witches and spirits live under ash trees, and in Poland people believe that witches gather under its branches for their meetings.[26] According to old Dutch lore, witches use a branch of ash wood when making their broomsticks.[27]

For all this, ash is widely used for protection against evil forces, particularly in France, where one regional custom says one should sew a sprig of ash with a little elm bark into the inside of one's jacket.[28] In the British Isles, the ash is always considered to have a benevolent force. Spenser writes that the ash is 'for nothing ill'—thus, for good.[29] And ash rods were used up until the nineteenth century to cure sick animals.[30] In the Scottish Highlands, when a baby was born a green stick of ash was placed in the fire; when it was hot some of the sap would leak out. When cool, this sap was placed on the baby's tongue.[31] Ash branches are used in charms and divinations, and the wood itself is used at Yule, when in some regions it is burned as the ashen faggot. Wassailing is an English winter custom, and an old Hampshire Yule song shows that the wassail cup was at least sometimes made of ash wood:

Wassail, wassail to our town,
The cup is white, the ale is brown;
The cup is made of ashen tree,
So is the ale of good barley.[32]

The following Yule 'drinking game' is particularly charming. In the farms and inns of Devon and Somerset, the Yule ashen faggot was burned when all were present at a festive evening. It was prepared as follows: bound with nine withies (slim branches) it is lit with charred twigs from the previous year's faggot. As it burns and as each band of withies bursts, those present take it in turns to make a toast, and everyone takes a swig of cider.[33]

A twig of ash with an even number of leaves has special powers. Such a twig is called an 'even ash' and is used in this Cornish luck charm: 'Even ash, I thee do pluck, hoping thus to meet good luck; if no luck I get from thee, I shall wish thee on the tree.'[34] The even ash is also used in a Somerset love spell: find a branch of ash with an even number of leaves, fold it in three and speak this charm before throwing it in the face of the person you would like to fall in love with you when you meet them next:

This even ash I double in three
The first one I meet my true love shall be.
If he be married let'n pass by,
But if he be single let'n draw nigh.[35]

Similar charms are found in Wiltshire, Yorkshire, Wales and other regions.[36]

∞   **Ash for protection.** Perform the French charm: sew a sprig of ash with a little elm bark into the inside of your coat or jacket.

∞   **Ash for luck.** Find a local ash tree, then look for a branch on which the number of leaves is even rather than odd. When you find one, repeat the Cornish luck charm and pluck it. We recommend giving an offering to the tree in thanks; milk, whiskey and cream are known to be received favourably.

19

∞ **Ash for love.** Perform the Somerset love spell above. On an ash tree in your neighbourhood, find a branch on which the number of leaves is even rather than odd. When you do find such a branch, ask the tree's blessing and pluck it, once you feel it has given you permission. Then fold the branch in three and throw it in the face of the person you want to fall in love with you the next time you see them. Admittedly, this unusual, sudden gesture may cause them some consternation.

∞ **Ash for the blessing of strength.** Perform the toasting game with an ash log at Yule, as outlined above. It is a 'game' played at party to which you invite your friends, to be held at a place with an open fireplace. Have plenty of alcoholic drinks ready, and prepare the log in advance.

∞ **Ash for animal wellbeing.** Make a wand of ash to use when doing spells involving animals, be they pets or wild species. This is especially suitable for pet owners, animal-lovers and veterinarians. To make a wand, first go to a local ash tree, ideally on a Wednesday, and ask its permission to cut a small branch. If the tree assents, cut a thin branch, making it the same length as the distance from your middle fingertip to your elbow. Peel the bark off immediately. Let it dry, then sand it. After a week, polish it with a mixture of oil and wax.

∞ **Ash for a baby blessing.** Put a dab of ash sap on the baby's tongue to grant it luck throughout its life. This requires a bit of planning, as first you need to find the nearest ash tree, then cut a twig from the growing tree at a time of year when the sap will flow freely from it. Finally, you need to get the baby to accept the ash sap. All in all, this is one of the more challenging baby blessings provided by the folklore record.

Balm

Also known as lemon balm, melissa
Melissa officinalis. Attribution: Jupiter (Culpeper), Sun (Lilly)
This is an important magical herb which gets much of its reputation from early physicians. Its foremost power is that it brings comfort, cheer, and—from there—energy for life. In southern Europe, its folk names include heart's delight and

the elixir of life. People have used it across the centuries. Ninth- and tenth-century Arab physicians prescribed it for people suffering from uneasiness and worry.[37] Gerard's herbal says that if you drink it in wine it 'drives away melancholy'. Culpeper says it is effective to 'expel those melancolly vapors from the Spirits'. In Shakespeare's plays, balm is used to assuage the king's sorrows.[38] Paracelsus asserted that the herb could completely revive a person who was unwell.[39]

Balm has a special relationship to bees. Both of lemon balm's given Greek names—*melissa* and the lesser-known name of *apiastrum*—mean 'bee'/'honey bee'. According to Pliny the Elder, bees were 'delighted with this herb above others'. In ancient Greece, sprigs of lemon balm were placed into beehives to attract wandering honeybee swarms. It is believed to keep them happy and more likely to stay rather than swarm away.[40]

∞ **Balm for happiness, against melancholy.** For melancholy, we recommend you prepare lemon-balm tea, ideally making it in a yellow or purple cup. Lemon balm can be incorporated into a spell for happiness: wrap a bunch of fresh sprigs in yellow and purple ribbons and place them at the centre of the arrangement. If you have only dried balm, put the dried, crumbled leaves into oil to infuse, then use the scented oil to anoint the person who is being treated. We highly recommend essential oil of lemon balm as a mood-lifter. Infuse it in water using an oil burner; the scent will permeate your home and change the atmosphere significantly.

∞ **Balm for bee blessing.** Use lemon-balm flowers, branches or oils in bee-keeping spells or bee-goddess rituals.

Basil

Ocimum basilicum. Attribution: Mars (Culpeper), Jupiter (Lilly)

Basil, a common kitchen herb, is nonetheless a plant associated with scorpions and basilisks. For ancient Greeks and Romans, it brings madness, misfortune, hatred and exhaustion. On Crete, putting basil on someone's windowsill brings a curse upon them.

Basil

In parts of Italy, basil goes by the name of little-love and kiss-me-Nicholas, names inviting sexual overtures. In Italian courting lore, basil is deemed to be full of sexual meaning: an unmarried woman wears it in her girdle (near her sexual organs); a married woman wears it upon her head (away from them). A man would go courting with a sprig of basil and place it upon the windowsill of his beloved; to place it directly into her hand would be disrespectful.[41] Sometimes, and in some places, basil is simply a sign of love. Italians of both sexes will give a little pot of basil to the person they are in love with or whom they consider very special.[42] In Romania, the maid who has set her cap at a young man will surely win his affection if she can get him to accept a sprig of basil from her hand. In Moldavia, too, if a man accepts a bit of basil from a lady, he will fall head over heels in love with her, to the point that she can control him utterly.

Basil became a symbol of tragic love in Renaissance Italy; for example, Giovanni Boccaccio used it to symbolise the tragic love between Lisabetta and Lorenzo in *The Decameron*. In Crete, the word for basil means 'love washed with tears'.[43] A Cretan folk song runs:

> Basil, herb of mourning,
> blossom in front of my little window;
> I, too, will go to sleep full of sorrow,
> and will fall asleep crying.[44]

It is a remarkable plant and there are very mixed beliefs about its powers; even Culpeper commented on the conflict of ideas about it.[45]

∽ **Basil for friendship.** Give someone you like a basil plant or basil sprig. Alternatively, make them a meal of pasta pesto; pesto is made with crushed basil leaves.

∽ **Basil for quick love.** Give the person you want to fall in love with a basil plant or a sprig of basil, or serve them a meal of pasta pesto.

Bay

Also known as laurel
Laurus nobilis. Attribution: Sun (Culpeper, Lilly)
This beautiful small tree with its aromatic leaves has featured in myth and legend since ancient times. The bay is the wood that nymph Daphne transformed into tree form. It was also the ancient Greeks' branch of honour and victory—Olympic winners were crowned with laurel, as were graduating doctors. In Rome, bay was used for crowns of Apollo, and the Muses are often crowned with laurel: thus, it signifies honour among poets.

Bay offers protection from evil. Greeks used the expression 'I carry a laurel stick' to show that they weren't afraid of witchcraft or poison.[46] In Western Europe across the centuries, it was thought that keeping a laurel leaf in your mouth granted you protection; Madame de Staël was said to do this.[47] Thomas Lupton, in his *Sixth Book of Notable Things* (dated c.1700) wrote, 'Neyther falling sicknes, neyther devyll, will infest or hurt one in that place where a Bay-tree is.'[48] In England, right up through the twentieth century, it was considered a tree of protection.[49]

Bay is a health-bringer: one of many examples is the ancient Greek custom of hanging sprigs over the door of a sick room to drive away evil spirits.[50] Culpeper writes, 'It is a tree of the Sun, and under the celestial sign Leo, and resisteth witchcraft very potently, as also all the evils old Saturn can do to the body of man, and they are not a few.'

It is also used to promote love: an old English charm for a couple to stay in love is that they pick a sprig of bay together then divide it and each keep their piece safe. So long as each keeps their half of the sprig, their love will stay strong.

In addition, bay is a herb of oracles. The Delphic oracle inhaled or chewed its leaves. Evelyn remarks that psychic people would sleep in the branches of the laurel tree or on mattresses of bay leaves; Juvenal alludes to this practice.[51] Evelyn adds that bay and chasteberry are herbs which 'greatly composed the phansy and did facilitate true visions, and that the first [bay] was specially efficacious to inspire a poetical fury'.[52]

Bay also has the power to bring back straying lovers; it is an old custom that to cause them to return, you simply need to burn bay leaves.

However, bay can be used for unkind purposes, too. A fifteenth-century spell from Germanic lands relates that to cause enmity one should take a bay leaf, divide it in two, write a name on each half, stitch them together with a needle and thread, then throw it into water.[53]

∞ **Bay for visions.** We recommend taking plenty of time if you wish to use bay to facilitate visions and psychic insights. For this, you need both dried and fresh bay leaves. Allocate an evening for the process, darken a cosy, warm space and put on gentle music, and after a hot bath settle down for a quiet, uninterrupted period of a few hours, ideally around an open fire, so you can gaze into the flickering flames. Do some yoga or breathing exercises, then burn two crushed dried bay leaves in a censer, so they smoulder like incense. Gently inhale the scented fumes, then chew one of the bay leaves. Drink warm water and rest, thinking relaxing thoughts. Write down the things that come into your mind in a notebook. At the end of the process, go to bed early and sleep as deeply as you can.

∞ **Bay for wellbeing.** Drink bay-leaf tea; simply pour boiling water into a mug over dried, crushed bay leaves, or over three fresh leaves. Bay is a solar plant, full of the forces of radiant wellbeing, so we recommend drinking the tea as part of a solar working—on a Sunday, using yellow crockery, or while wearing any gold jewellery you may own. While drinking the tea, we like to burn bay leaves as incense.

∞ **Bay for love.** Perform the English love spell above to help a couple stay together. On a Friday, the day of love, pick a bay leaf, then divide it in two. Place each half on a piece of card to keep it flat and put it in a small envelope. You may wish to write on the cards or envelopes—perhaps the lovers' initials, and/or a Venus seal or sigil; these are easily found online, under 'Key of Solomon Venus'. Give one of the envelopes to both partners in the couple with strict instructions that they are to keep it safe. A simple way to do this is to keep it under their side of the mattress or in their bedside cabinet.

∽ **Bay to bring a lover back.** This is done by burning bay leaves. We recommend doing this on a Friday night, ideally in the days leading up to the full moon, when the moon is growing. As in all such workings, we caution careful consideration of the necessity—and the advisability—of pursuing such a course of action.[54]

∽ **Bay for protection.** Carry a bay leaf or include bay leaves in your spell bags. Alternatively, grow a bay tree inside your house or near the front door. We recommend crumbling a few bay leaves into a hot bath. This makes the bathing experience aromatically calming and enlivening; sometimes we supplement the leaves with a few drops of bay essential oil.

∽ **Bay for honour and fame.** Use bay leaves for success in competitive sport and also in medicine. You can also use it for spells to bring success in music, drama and literary careers. The best day for doing such spells is Sunday, the day of the Sun, the force of success, of wellbeing and winning.

∽ **Bay in magic to cause enmity.** Perform the fifteenth-century German spell above. As with all matters where one feels a need to create disharmony or enmity, it is essential to first spend time assessing your motives and weighing up your decision carefully, in line with your ethics and highest moral standards.

Beech
Genus *Fagus*. Attribution: Saturn (Culpeper), Jupiter (Lilly)
The beech, in Somerset folklore, is deemed to be a holy tree, a tree of pure goodness and protection. People are told that if they get lost in the woods, they should find shelter under a beech, because once they are under its branches, nothing can get close enough to harm them. If you pray under a beech tree, your prayers will go straight to heaven. The tree

is offended if people use bad language in its presence; when they do, the beech rustles its leaves or drops a branch.[55] It is used for protection in some regions, too: if you write the letter 'T' on a beech leaf, it will keep you safe from the evil eye for as long as you carry it on you.[56]

∽　**Beech for urgent prayers.** Find the nearest beech tree and make your petitions under its branches. First, however, be sure your conscience is clear and your heart is pure, carrying out rites of purification if necessary. Then, give thanks to the tree and make it an offering, asking kindly for its blessing and help. Only then should you commence your petitions for your own urgent needs.

∽　**Beech for personal protection.** Find a beech tree, ideally one in your neighbourhood. Introduce yourself, make an offering and ask the tree's blessing. Then pick a leaf, write the letter 'T' on it, and put it into a small bag or envelope and carry it with you.

Betony

Also known as wood betony, bishopswort
Genus *Stachys*.[57] Attribution: Jupiter (Culpeper, Lilly)
Betony is a common wild plant with delicate purple flowers. It is very much a plant of magic workers, too: in early Germany, a witch was defined as 'she who digs up the betony'.[58]

According to the ancient Roman medical writer Antonius Musa, betony is effective against witchcraft attacks. It seems that everyone in Europe thought so, too; it was one of the most important herbs in Anglo-Saxon medicine to stop 'frightful nocturnal goblins and terrible sights and dreams'.[59] This belief continued into the later Middle Ages, when graveyards would be planted with betony to keep ghost activity down.

Betony is used magically to banish inner demons, too: anxiety, panic and depression. The early modern German writer Erasmus suggests that people hang betony around their neck as an amulet or charm if they need protection from 'fearful visions', adding that it is highly effective at 'driving away devils and despair'.[60] This spell from seventeenth-century London is in a similar vein.

Arthur Gauntlet's Sanity Spell

First, shave the person's head. Then take some betony and press it against the whole of the scalp ('the mould of the head'). Take a piece of cheese and write on it 'ANTABRAGON TETRAGRAMMATON', then give the cheese to the sufferer to eat. The person will recover from their mental suffering.[61]

Across the British Isles and Europe, betony's magical power to relieve mental distress is found again and again. An old Welsh sleep charm says that to prevent (unpleasant) dreaming, you should hang betony leaves around your neck before going to bed. An alternative is to drink betony juice just before lying down to sleep.[62]

∽   **Betony against anxiety and despair.** You can use betony in any number of ways—it is so versatile. Wear it around your neck, drink betony tea, or keep betony as a house plant. We recommend betony-leaf tea, which has long been drunk in Britain as a substitute for normal black tea. Dry the leaves, then pour boiling water over them to make a refreshing drink with special powers against anxiety and despair. We advise doing any work with betony on a Thursday, the day of wellbeing and expansive good fortune, which shares the same potencies as the betony plant itself.

∽   **Betony against nightmares.** Choose from the ways of using betony above. We recommend keeping the plant or the dried herb under your pillow or under the bed. Wrap it in purple cloth or with a purple ribbon; this is the colour of Jove, who is happy and content—hence the word 'jovial'.

∽   **Betony against melancholy.** Perform Arthur Gauntlet's sanity spell above, modifying it as necessary.

Birch

Genus *Betula*. Attribution: Venus (Culpeper), Jupiter (Lilly)
The birch is widely called upon for protection in many parts of Europe and England. Branches, twigs and boughs are placed at windows and doors to keep out misfortune and to avert the evil eye. To give just one example, in Herefordshire

on May Day, people used to tie red and white ribbons to birch trunks and branches then set them outside their barns to protect the animals within throughout the year to come.[63] On the Scottish isle of Colonsay, it is a custom to protect babies from misfortune by hanging a bundle of birch twigs over the cradle.[64]

Birch is the tree of courting and love in Wales. It was traditional to go courting among birches, courtship items are made of birch wood and wreaths of birch were woven as love tokens. A Welsh 'broomstick wedding' was always done over a broom 'made of silver birch wood'.[65]

Coleridge wrote of 'Most beautiful of forest trees, the Lady of the Woods'. The idea struck a chord, and the phrase 'lady of the woods' persists in English lore. Coleridge tapped into a feeling which is recognised in other regions; for example, the Russians call the birch 'The Lady of the Forest'.[66] In Russia, birch trees, one of the earliest to blossom in springtime, were the centre of a young women's woodland ritual known as 'Semik' in which the maidens dressed and bent the birches to channel life energies.[67]

Russian Spell for Lost Items

This is traditionally used for lost livestock, and is a letter to the spirit of the woods, the *leshii*. Get some birch bark. Write from right to left on it, in triplicate. The opening address is 'I write to the tsar of the forest, the tsaritsa of the forest and their little children; to the tsar of the earth ..., to the tsar of the water ... I inform you that ...' State your name and the lost items and kindly petition them to return them if they have them. Politeness is important. Place a copy in the following three places: tied to a tree, tied to a stone which you then throw into water, and buried in the earth. The items will reappear.[68]

The legendary Russian witch Baba Yaga has a broomstick made of silver birch, which reinforces our sense that, in Russia, the tree has a special connection to women.[69] In Somerset, the birch tree is considered a tree of witches; they believe witches cut their brooms from birch. As a result, it is there considered a tree of evil. In Taunton, a ghostly spirit woman haunts travellers on the darkened road; white, skinny and terrifying, she is 'The One with the White Hand', and one account identifies her explicitly as the birch tree's spirit.[70]

∾ **Birch for love.** Give items of birchwood to the one you love. Birch is sometimes used to make wooden spoons. We think that a large birchwood spoon is the ideal magical love gift; it is an exceptionally magical item. In Wales, it is customary for sweethearts to give one another spoons as love tokens.

∾ **Birch for house protection and blessing.** Place birch twigs or branches above doors and windows.

∾ **Birch for a magic tool.** Make a besom (rough broom), cutting your own birch twigs for the brush.

∾ **Birch for a baby blessing.** Make a birch-twig bundle to place in a corner of the baby's room. The bundle can include other baby-blessing herbs (listed at the beginning of this book), in order to make an attractive mixed bundle. We suggest using a red ribbon to tie the bundle, as red is the colour of vitality and life itself.

Bog myrtle

Myrica gale. Attribution: none given in either Culpeper or Lilly
This strongly aromatic plant is well known and loved in Scotland, though it grows across all of North-western Europe. In the Scottish Highlands, bog myrtle is used against the evil eye. A person who has been the victim of the evil eye ('overlooked') is pushed through a large hoop of bog myrtle and this undoes the curse.[71] Such a hoop should be the size of a hula hoop or a bit larger.

∾ **Bog myrtle for personal protection.** Do this in circumstances where you know that someone thinks ill of you, particularly if they are envious of you. You will probably do several things to protect yourself, but as part of a ritual or set of actions, we suggest that you sit or stand in the centre of a ring of bog-myrtle leaves. To perform the working as the Scots themselves do, make a hoop of myrtle with a circumference of approximately 5 or 6 feet and ceremoniously step through it.

Borage
Also known as starflower
Borago officinalis. Attribution: Jupiter (Culpeper, Lilly)
Borage is a herb that has long been used in magic; great power is universally attributed to it. It was eaten for courage by Roman soldiers before they went into battle, and its reputation for bestowing courage continued across the centuries. Medieval knights wore scarves embroidered with borage flowers for the same reason, and it was also sometimes taken in wine or beer. In the seventeenth century, Gerard the herbalist related a well-known saying: 'I, borage, bring always courage.' Edmund Gayton wrote in his 1659 book, *Art of Longevity:*

> Have you no courage?
> At any time revive your soul with Borage ...
> Sirrup of Borage will make sad men glad
> And the same sirrup doth restore the mad.

In addition to courage, borage brings happiness. The eleventh-century School of Salerno says, 'When talking of Borage, this much is clear/It warms the heart and brings good cheer.'[72] In early modern England, it was used to lift melancholy. Burton, in his *Anatomy of Melancholy*, wrote that borage was 'against this malady [melancholy] most frequently prescribed'. Gerard prescribed a borage salad to help patients feel joy. Culpeper, similarly, wrote that 'the leaves are good to expel pensiveness and melancholy'.

Borage can be prepared for use in any number of ways. It is effective 'whether in substance, juice, roots, seeds, flowers, leaves, decoctions, distilled waters, extracts, oyles &c'. It can be taken 'in Broth, in Wine, in Conserves, Syrops, &c'. Its flowers 'cheer the hard student'. Culpeper recommends that 'candied or jellied flowers comfort the heart and spirits of those who are sick from passions of the heart'. Most useful, however, is the borage recipe of the Countess of Kent (1582–1651), included in her collection of remedies.

30

Lady Elizabeth Grey's 'Excellent Syrrup against Melancholy'

Take four quarts of the juice of Pearmains, and twice as much of the juice of Bugloss and Borage, if they be gotten, a drachm of the best English Saffron, bruise it, and put it into the juice, then take two drachms of Kermes [a red dye] small beaten to powder, mix it also with the juice; so being mixt, put them into an earthen vessel, covered or stopt forty-eight hours, then strain it and allow a pound of sugar to every quart of juice, and so boil it to the ordinary weight of a syrrup, after it is boiled, take one drachm of the spices of Dramber, and two dracms of the spices of Diamargariton frigidum [powder of pearl], and so sew the same slenderly in a linnen bag, that you may put the same easily into the bottle of syrrup, and so let it hang with a thred out at the mouth of the bottle, the spices must be put into the surrup in the bag: so soon as the syrrup is off the fire, whilst it is hot, then afterwards put it into the bottle, and there let it hang: put but a spoonful or two of Honey amongst it, whilst it is boiling, and it will make the scum rise, and the syrrup very clear. You must add to it the quantity of a quarter of a pint of juice of Balm.[73]

The herbalist Gerard also suggested syrup of borage flowers to 'purgeth melancholy and quieteth the phreneticke and lunaticke person'. Such a syrup as this would be employed for psychological disturbance, as well as depression.

∽ **Borage for courage.** Eat bits of the borage plant in any way you like for courage, but if you have time, we recommend making borage soup, adding a sprinkling of chili pepper or black pepper to it, as these are the seasonings of martial power, as Mars symbolises warrior energy. There are any number of wonderful borage soup recipes online. If you have the option, make this a ceremonial meal on a Tuesday, serving it in a red bowl or on a red tablecloth.

∽ **Borage for happiness, against depression.** Make and drink an improvised version of the syrup outlined above. An alternative is to make and eat candied borage flowers. The internet has simple instructions on easy methods to make candied borage flowers. For a friend suffering from melancholy, there is no nicer magical gift than a box of home-made candied borage flowers.

∞ **Borage to cure heartbreak.** As above.

∞ **Borage against anxiety and mental unrest.** Take borage in any form, but we particularly recommend borage syrup for anxiety, and we like to prepare and eat an old English traditional salad of cucumber and borage (recipes can be found online). Cucumber is a lunar plant, and therefore soothing and cooling.

Box

Buxus sempervirens. Attribution: not given by Culpeper; Saturn [Lilly]

A bushy low tree with tiny, shiny dark green leaves, box is often used to make hedges at the borders of English gardens. In some parts of northern Europe (northern France, the Netherlands and Belgium), it was the custom to use box branches to serve as local substitutes for the traditional palm branches of Palm Sunday; for this reason, they became known as 'palms'. In these areas, the box tree was understood to have the power to deter demons from houses. In Limburg in the sixteenth century, there was a custom of carving amulets from box wood to wear around the neck to protect the wearer from evil magic; if a person was thought to be cursed, they would be given a drink made from box, and when they had drunk it, the spell would be undone.[74]

∞ **Box for personal protection.** Carve a small amulet from box wood and wear it around your neck.

∞ **Box for undoing a spell.** Prepare a drink from box and drink it. You can make traditional Turkish box tea by pouring boiling water over a few box leaves.

Broom

Cytisus scoparius. Attribution: Mars (Culpeper)

This yellow-flowered wild shrub is very much a witch's plant. Broom tops are known to be used by witches as their flying besoms (broomsticks). Like many plants associated with supernatural beings, it should not be brought into the house in May. A traditional Sussex rhyme runs, 'Sweep the house with blessed broom in May/Sweep the head of the household away.'[75]

∞   **Broom plant in ritual practice.** Create a ritual or spell in which the broom tops symbolise brooms on which you fly to other realms.

Butterwort

Pinguicula vulgaris. Attribution: given in neither Culpeper nor Lilly

This fen-growing herb with purple flowers is a plant which has powers of protection. It is revered especially in Scotland. In the Inner Hebrides, people make butterwort butter and give it to their children to keep them safe from the fairies. Carrying a sprig of butterwort keeps you safe from supernatural witches and from all ill:

> From all despite,
> From the sorrow of love ungiven,
> From a foeman's stroke,
> From the gnaw of hunger,
> Or from drowning, the doom of the sea.[76]

∞   **Butterwort for a baby blessing.** Make butterwort butter for parents as a 'magical' blessing for the whole family when a baby is born. This is made simply by finely chopping a couple of the thick, fleshy leaves then mixing them into soft butter. Form the butter into a pat or put it into a ramekin or a butter mould and chill in the fridge. Wrapped in foil or baking paper and tied with a ribbon, it makes a lovely good-luck gift for new parents.

∞ **Butterwort for protection.** Carry a sprig of butterwort on you and involve it in spells. We suggest reciting the above poem when picking it or using it.

Bryony, white
Also known as English mandrake and ladies' seal
Bryonia alba. Attribution: Mars (Culpeper)
Bryony is an English plant that grows wild, and its main magical use is as a substitute for mandrake; it became such a standard substitute that it was sometimes called 'English mandrake'. It is the roots of mandrake—and thus bryony—that are used; they resemble those of humans. In 1568, William Turner, Dean of Wells, wrote, 'The rootes which are counterfited and made like little pupettes or mammettes which come to be sold in England in boxes with heir and such forme as a man hath [i.e. genitals].'[77]

You can find and dig up the bryony root to use in carving a spell poppet (doll). However, be careful, as the spirit of the plant is prickly and protective. To dig it up will bring you bad luck, so it may not be worth it. 'In December 1908, a man employed in digging a neglected garden half a mile from Stratford upon Avon cut a large root of white bryony through with his spade. He called it mandrake, and ceased to work at once, saying it was "awful bad luck". Before the week was out, he fell down some steps and broke his neck.'[78]

∞ **Bryony in spells.** Carve the root into the shape of the person you are working the magic upon and use this poppet as their 'stand-in'. It is suggested that you mark or carve the bryony root in some way to indicate the person's identity: shape it with their features, inscribe their initials, tie it with a strand of their hair, or something similar.

Caper spurge
Also known as mole plant, springwort; medieval name: virgin's milk
Euphorbia lathyris. Attribution: none given in either Culpeper or Lilly
This is a tall weed which grows on waste ground. It is used infrequently in magic, but is one of the plants traditionally

gathered on St John's Eve, or Midsummer's Eve. Leaves, flowers and branches gathered then have the most power. Folklore says that one should seek out caper spurge during the night of St John's Eve, searching for plants that are near ferns. If you find some, collect them, dry and save. The great power of caper spurge is the power to magically open locks. Even better, it can find hidden doorways and cause them to open.[79] Like many St John's Eve plants, it gives protection from witchcraft attacks: Jersey folklore specifically recommends growing a plant of caper spurge in the garden to protect everyone who lives in the house.[80] All parts of the plant, including the seeds and the roots, are poisonous, so do not eat any part of it.

∞ **Caper spurge for protection**. Plant caper spurge in or near your house. If a friend is moving into a new home, a caper spurge plant is an ideal housewarming gift.

∞ **Caper spurge for opening closed doorways.** Use the dried herb for this. You can use the herb in a potion both to unlock literal doors and to gain access to institutions and meetings which are gate-kept. For example, you can use caper spurge in a spell to be accepted into a university programme or to be sent an invitation to a private event. In any situation where there is a virtual door you cannot open, caper spurge will assist you. Wave a branch of caper spurge at your laptop as you send off a related email, or as you send a letter through the post. Another method is to lay caper-spurge stems around an item symbolising the place you want to enter. We advise doing this on a Wednesday and then lighting an orange candle next to the arrangement. Orange is the colour of mercurial force, which opens pathways quickly.

Caraway
Carum carvi. Attribution: Mercury (Culpeper)
In modern times, caraway is known as a cooking herb, but in the Middle Ages women would sew caraway seeds into the clothing of their beloved to keep them faithful while they were away on Crusade.

∞ **Caraway for faithfulness.** Slip caraway seeds into the clothing of your lover or spouse to keep them from straying. As they are small and unobtrusive, caraway seeds are easily used for this purpose. A few seeds can be added, too, to your sweetheart's luggage before they go on a solo trip.

Catnip

Also known as catmint, nep

Nepeta cataria. Attribution: Venus/Mars (Culpeper)[81]

This herb, famous for being the delight of cats, is now available in every pet store. It has magical powers, not recreational ones, for humans. Catnip has the power to turn even the most gentle person into someone fierce and quarrelsome. It is also a plant to give courage; legend tells of a famed French hangman who could not bear to execute his duties unless he had chewed some catnip root.[82]

∞ **Catnip for courage.** Locate dried catnip root, or prepare your own, ideally doing so on a Tuesday and leaving the root on a red-coloured plate. When you do a spell for extra courage to help you carry out an especially difficult task, eat a small portion of the root, too.

∞ **Catnip to create conflict.** Sprinkle catnip around a meeting place if you wish to arouse discord among the people who will assemble there. If you wish to make someone angry, put some catnip near them. This might be by their bed, at their work station or in their pocket. We urge caution and restraint in cases where you are tempted to use the plant in this way; it is advisable to first undertake a period of self-reflection to assess your motivation and ethics, considering what is likely to be the best way forward in the longer term.

Chamomile

Genus *Asteraceae*. Attribution: Sun (Culpeper)

This delicate-looking herb, which has hundreds of tiny white flowers, grows low on the ground like a grass, so in England it used to be popular to grow it in lawns. It comes in two main varieties: Roman (English chamomile) and German (wild chamomile). They are related and resemble one another, and they have the same magical attributes. One of the old names for chamomile was earth-apple, due to the flowers having apple-like scent.

Chamomile is one of the most important herbs in the magical pharmacopeia, being one of the St John's herbs, those which custom says should be gathered on Midsummer's Day.[83] People hang a wreath of chamomile on their door on St John's Day to protect the house from misfortune in the coming season.[84] In an old German custom, farmers' wives would hang chamomile inside the house; if an evil-wisher came into the home, the chamomile would start to sway and swish, giving the home-owner a red alert about this person. They would be trouble, however pleasant and genuine they might seem.[85]

In British lore, chamomile embodies resilience: 'A camomile bed, the more it is trodden, the more it will spread.'[86] In Tudor England, chamomile was a plant of humility and patience.[87] This humility and patience, however, is underpinned by great resilience, which will ultimately make it triumph over adversity.

∞ **Chamomile for house protection.** Put chamomile in a house-protection wreath and hang it on your front door. The herbs for house protection are listed at the front of this book, and a combination of them in a wreath makes an attractive and effective gift for a friend moving into a new home, or simply to bless a home which has been through a time of trouble.

∞ **Chamomile for detecting bad people.** Hang chamomile in your house near the door and it will alert you when you have a guest with negative energies. We suggest using chamomile in the same way in your work space; you can hang a ribbon-wrapped sprig from the corner of a computer monitor, or have a small bouquet of dried chamomile flowers in a tiny vase on your desk.

∞ **Chamomile for resilience and endurance.** Use chamomile in spells to give someone the ability to bounce back from knock-backs or from situations where they are repeatedly put down. We recommend giving the person a potted chamomile plant. Alternatively, advise them to drink a cup of chamomile tea each evening for a week. If you are doing a spell, we recommend that you use a small fabric bundle filled with chamomile to represent the victim, or else a poppet with chamomile stuffing.

Chasteberry

Also known as chaste tree, monk's pepper, agnus castus, vitex *Agnus Castus*. Attribution: none given in either Culpeper or Lilly This shrub grows in Mediterranean regions and has been used in magic and medicine across Europe for centuries. If drunk or imbibed, it promotes prophecy and clairvoyance. John Evelyn says that it 'greatly composed the phansy and did facilitate true visions'.[88]

Chasteberry is most famous, however, for its connection with chastity and its power to help one suppress lustful desire.[89] Even in myth, it is a herb of decorum, matronliness and wifeliness. In Greek myth, Hera was born under a chasteberry tree. Pliny wrote, 'the Athenian matrons preserving their chastity at the Thesmophoria strew their beds with its leaves'. In Rome, vestal virgins carried bunches of chasteberry twigs as a symbol of chastity. Later, under Christianity, novices entering a monastery would walk down a path strewn with chasteberry blossom to confirm their chastity—a ritual that continues to the present day in some parts of Italy.[90] Robert Chester's 1601 poem 'Love's Martyr' puts it poetically:

> [The poet says] Of Agnus Castus speak a word or two.
> [Nature replies, saying:] That I shall I briefly;
> It is the very handmaid to Vesta, or to perfect Chastity.
> The hot inflamed spirit is allayed
> By this sweet herb that bends to Luxury,
> It drieth up the seed of Venery:
> The leaves being laid upon the sleepers bed,
> With chastness, cleanness, pureness he is fed.

Gerard, the seventeenth-century English herbalist, prescribed the herb medicinally to help people refrain from having sex.[91]

∞   **Chasteberry for calming passion.** Use in spells to calm
unruly romantic and sexual obsessions. We recommend doing
such spells on Saturdays or Mondays and taking the chasteberry as a tea. In the spell to calm infatuation, you can dip a
photograph of yourself and one of the object of your desire
into a bowl of cool chasteberry tea.

∞   **Chasteberry for supernatural abilities.** If you wish
to enhance your psychic powers, make and drink a tea of
chasteberry leaves, but be warned: the tea does not taste
wonderful. Tea drinking can form part of a more elaborate
occasion, in which you lay out soft cushions, dim the lights,
put on soft music or play a drum. You can set out a crystal
ball or a pendulum to use once you are deeply relaxed. We
always recommend making these special nights on the full
moon, which is the night of heightened psychic power each
month.

Chervil

Anthriscus cerefolium. Attribution: Jupiter (Culpeper)
Chervil is an aromatic herb grown in medieval gardens and
is used widely in French cooking. It resembles a more delicate version of flatleaf parsley and has a mild, sweet aniseed flavour. It is not widely used for magic, but an English
magical folk grimoire says that if you're in danger of being
cursed, you should carry this herb around and you will be
free of it.[92]

∞   **Chervil for protection.** Carry a little bunch of chervil
on you as you go about your day. We recommend making a
little bundle of it tied with gold or yellow string then putting
it in a small bag to carry in your pocket or handbag. You
can perform a small ritual at your home for a friend who is
vulnerable or under attack, to give them the blessing of protection: invite them over, then take a bunch of chervil and
use it as a sprinkler to sprinkle them with saltwater. Then,
chop up the chervil bunch and add it to the meal you are
cooking them. We have done this, using tasty chervil recipes
found online.

Chicory

Cichorium intybus. Attribution: Jupiter (Culpeper)

This common wild plant, found in verges and overgrown areas, is notable for its bright blue flowers and slightly woody stems. It has few uses in folk magic, but we have found one, from England. A late-sixteenth-century text says it has the power to attract beneficence from those who hold power, 'a thing which superstition hath believed, that the body anoynted with the juice of chicory is very available to obtain the favour of great persons'.[93] It also has the power to open locked doors on 25 July: on that day, use a golden knife to cut the plant in silence, then hold it against the keyhole, still without uttering a word, for if you speak it is believed you will die; if you do this successfully, the locked door will open.[94]

∾ **Chicory for gaining patronage or favours from powerful people.** Crush the chicory, release the juice and smear it on your body. Do this before you go into a meeting with the person whose favour you need or want. If you are not meeting the person in question but are corresponding with them, smear yourself with chicory before sending a letter or composing an email. In addition to anointing yourself with chicory juice, we suggest wearing some item of clothing which is purple, to bring out the Jupiterian qualities of the plant and the situation. Jupiter's colour purple has the power of being placed in good favour by powerful people and institutions.

∾ **Chicory for opening locked doors.** On 25 July, make a point of cutting some chicory in silence, with a golden cutting edge, if you can find one. Place it, in silence, against whatever 'keyhole' there is to the place that is closed to you. We recommend using this spell for gaining access to places and institutions that are hard to enter. For example, applying to a selective university course, a job for which there is a lot of competition, or membership of a club with strict criteria. Your keyhole representative could be an image of the place, a student card or a membership card: something that serves as 'admission' to that place in daily life.

Cinquefoil

Also known as the five-leaved herb; American name: five-finger grass.

Genus *Potentilla*. Attribution: Jupiter (Culpeper), Sun (Lilly)

Cinquefoil is rarely used in British and European folk magic, but in America it is widely employed in the hoodoo, or 'conjure', tradition. The plant's distinguishing feature is its five-leaved appearance, hence its English folk name, five-leaved herb, and the American five-finger grass. It is not entirely absent from English folk traditions, however, for Northumberland lore holds that if you wear a crown of cinquefoil, you will see fairies.[95] Cinquefoil is found in the famed French folk-magic guidebook, the Book of Secrets of Albertus Magnus, which says 'it giveth abundance of eloquence, if he have it with him, and he shall obtain it that he desireth'.[96]

❧ **Cinquefoil for gaining favours.** Carry it with you when you go to speak to a person of power to ask something of them, and you will get what you ask for. We recommend making a little bundle bound with ribbons or fabric in the colours orange and purple. Orange is mercurial, the colour of smooth talk and eloquence, while purple is the colour of benevolence from people of great power. If you can choose the day for such a meeting, we urge you to try for a Wednesday or a Thursday.

❧ **Cinquefoil to see fairies.** Make a crown of cinquefoil and go to a local spot which is said to house fairies. Leaf crowns are easily made with the help of kitchen twist-ties or florist's wire. We suggest making your outing on a full moon or, even better, a night of supernatural power, such as Midsummer's Eve or May Eve. To find fairies in your local area, look for wooded places where few people go—see if there is a grove of elm or walnut trees, or a lone hawthorn tree.

Cloves

Syzygium aromaticum. Attribution: Jupiter (Lilly)

Cloves are not native to Europe but grow in what used to be called the Spice Islands. They have been present in Britain and Europe since the Middle Ages due to trade with Asia;

since then, they have been used in meat preserving. Cloves appear only rarely in the folk spells in of Europe, but we have found two instances. In Portugal, a string of beaded cloves is put around a baby's neck to keep it safe from evil influences.[97] And Swedish bridegrooms sew cloves, garlic and rosemary into their wedding suit to keep away trolls and sprites.

∞   **Clove for a baby blessing.** Use clove in a magical protection charm for a baby. The Portuguese tradition of the clove necklace is not advisable in its traditional form, as necklaces on babies are a hazard. We recommend instead a blessing bag including cloves to be hung in a corner of the baby's room. Another alternative is a woven hoop of cloves, made to your own specification, which can serve as a room decoration or a window ornament near the baby, but safely out of reach.

∞   **Clove for bridegroom blessing (wedding).** Use clove in a spell or in a fabric wrap or small bag to give blessing and protection to a bridegroom for his marriage.

Clover, four-leaf

Genus *Trifolium*.[98] Attribution: Mercury (Culpeper)
Four-leafed clovers are among the most important plants of European magic and are the subject of hundreds of customs and gems of magical lore. It is universally recognised that they bring good fortune. The Gospelles of Dystaues (1507) say that,

> he that fyndeth the trayvle [trefoil, i.e. clover] with foure leues, and kepe it in reuerence knowe, for also true as the gospel yt he shall be ryche all his life.'[99]

If you carry it, you will happen upon good things in your path. 'If a man walking in the fields, find any four-leafed grasse, he shall in a small while after finde some good thing.'[100] Magic-workers have long treasured it and used it as an ingredient in their spells.

> I'll seek a four-leaved clover
> In all the fairy dells

And if I find the charmed leaf,
    Oh how I'll weave my spells.[101]

In the pre-modern era, when milkmaids placed bunches of grass on their heads to steady the milk-pails they carried there, some would sometimes see fairies and not understand why this had come about: the grass bunch, examined, would always reveal a four-leafed clover. Similar things happened in Ireland.[102] This trick can be worked deliberately, of course, and often was. Some people used to wear a crown of clover, with four-leafed clovers in it, in order to see the fairies; this was a custom in Northumberland.[103] A Cornwall account of 1881 relates that a man placed a green ointment on his eyes in order to see fairies, using four-leaved clover gathered 'at a certain time of the moon'.[104]

The clover ointment also makes the wearer invisible—in the same account, a man used the ointment to shoplift undetected in Penzance market.[105] The ability to see invisible beings such as fairies is also said to improve the ability to discern lies and perceive liars. A traditional English custom says that if you hold a four-leafed clover in your hand you will see right through illusions, and you will also see witches and sorcerers.[106] In Scotland, people believe that if you are speaking with someone who wishes to curse you or do magic against you, you will know it clearly if you are holding a four-leaf clover in your hand.[107]

Another power of the four-leaf clover is to bring lovers back and to keep them faithful. It is an old custom that when lovers are to be parted through travel, the lover staying behind places a four-leaf clover in the shoe of their departing sweetheart to ensure they come back, faithful and safe.[108] It is generally understood that a clover in the shoe is good luck for any traveller: they will be safe on their journey.[109]

Clover is also attributed with the power to help a person avoid military service.[110] It is lucky for gamblers, too, so long as they follow these rules: keep it on you always, never boast of it and never give it away.

∾ **Clover to see fairies (method 1).** Make a Northumbrian fairy crown: in simple terms, this consists of making a wreath

43

and inserting a four-leafed clover in it. Making flower and leaf crowns is a perfect activity for a weekend afternoon around the full moon. Invite a couple of friends over to drink herbal teas, eat cake and make the crowns. Have to hand some twist ties or a reel of florist's wire; these will hold your crown together. When affixing the clovers, however, be sure everyone present has stopped speaking. Folk magic generally requires that important moments of engagement with spirits are conducted in silence.

∽   **Clover to see fairies (method 2).** Make the Cornish ointment: use a four-leafed clover to make an ointment, plucking the clover at 'a certain time of the moon'; my tip is to gather it at full moon. To make an ointment, we recommend following the instructions of one of the many online videos available. An ointment is a simple creation, however. First, cut up a bunch of clover leaves and simmer them in a small pan in half an inch of water. Mash them every few minutes, until the water is very green and the leaves are part cooked. Then remove the mashed clover and simmer the green water until you have only about a teaspoonful left. Add 4 tablespoons of oil and 1 tablespoon of beeswax and mix until fully blended. Pour the mixture out into a small dish or sterile jar and let it cool.

∽   **Clover for safe travel.** Put a four-leaf clover in your shoe. If you have a friend who is going on a long journey, a four-leaf clover makes a perfect gift.

∽   **Clover for good luck in gambling and risk-taking.** Carry the clover with you, making sure to keep it on you always and ensuring that you never boast of it and never give it away. This will bring you good winnings when you play games of chance. Equally, it will be beneficial when you are taking risks as an entrepreneur.

∽   **Clover to detect lies.** Use a four-leaved clover if you want to see the truth of a situation, to see past someone's lies, or to perceive if someone wishes you ill, even if they seem to be treating you well. Hold it in your hand while you

are talking to them and you will perceive clearly any decep-
tion. Alternatively, place the clover under your pillow and ask
the plant to reveal the truth to you as you sleep or meditate,
then rest deeply, being open to any messages that may come
through. We recommend collecting your own clover, if possible, particularly if there is a matter that is concerning you
deeply.

∾   **Clover to detect malice or curses.** Use the method for
detecting lies above.

∾   **Clover for faithfulness.** When your sweetheart is going
away, put a four-leaf clover in his or her shoe, or in their
wallet or handbag. If you do this, they will return from their
trip having stayed loyal to you.

∾   **Clover to avoid military service.** Use a four-leaf clover
in a spell to avoid conscription. Such a spell should be done
with white tools, fabrics and dressings.

Clubmoss

Also known as ground pine, cloth-of-gold
Genus *Lycopodiacece*. Mars (Culpeper), Saturn along with all
mosses (Lilly)
Club moss or ground pine is a common, ground-hugging plant
which spreads web-like across the forest floor or through
shaded lawn grass; it has pine-like nibs with miniature needles
sticking out of them. One species, the fir club moss selago
(*Huperzia selago*), is the subject of a most remarkable tale.
Pliny specified that it was a valuable herb, to be gathered barefoot, with feet washed, while clad in white, after one had offered a sacrifice of bread and wine.[111] Winwood Reade relates
a fabulated account, based on a conflation of Pomponios Mela
and Pliny, of moon-worshipping druid priestesses on the isle of
Sena (now Saine, possibly Sein) on the Loire River:

> It was one of their rites to procure a virgin and to strip
> her naked, as an emblem of the moon in an unclouded
> sky. Then they sought for the wondrous selago or golden
> herb. She who pressed it with her foot slept, and heard the

language of animals. If she touched it with iron, the sky grew dark and a misfortune fell upon a world. When they had found it [the selago plant], the virgin traced a circle round it, and covering her hand in a white linen cloth which had never been before used, rooted it out with a point of her little finger—a symbol of the crescent moon. Then they washed it in a running spring, and having gathered green branches plunged into a river and splashed the virgin, who was thus supposed to resemble the moon clouded with vapors. When they retired, the virgin walked backwards that the moon might not return upon its path in the plain of the heavens.[112]

People in Brittany use selago (which they call 'cloth of gold') for magical purposes: they believe it gives a person the ability to understand the language of animals and birds, but in order for it to work, the person must cut it ceremoniously, without using metal.[113] In Scotland, club moss is used in medicinal remedies, for which it is collected ritually: 'on the third day of the moon, when the thin crescent is seen for the first time, show it the knife, with which the moss is to be cut', and address a charm to the plant.[114] Clubmoss is a magical protection herb as well as a medicine. An old Scottish charm says that if you carry clubmoss on you, you will be protected from misfortune.[115]

∞   **Clubmoss for protection.** Determine the third day after the next new moon (you can do this easily by looking online). Find a nearby clubmoss plant. On that night, go out either barefoot in a white robe, or fully naked. When you get to the plant, place a bit of bread and a few drops of red wine on the ground by it as an offering. Speak kindly to it, telling it your worries and asking it to bless you and keep you. Then pinch off a sprig, using your fingers. Wash it in fresh water and place it in a fabric wrap or sachet/bag. Carry it with you.

∞   **Clubmoss for animal communication.** For veterinarians, animal-shelter workers and pet owners, this is a wonderful charm. The collection of the clubmoss must be done correctly, however, for it to work well. We suggest using the method outlined in the preceding paragraph, but if you do a simpler version, remember that it is essential to cut the sprig without metal and to make an offering and speak to the plant. Once you have collected your clubmoss, prepare it to aid the person in animal communication. We suggest putting a few pinches of clubmoss in a bath, then giving the person some meditation time, during which the room is filled with clubmoss incense so they breathe the essence of the moss in deeply. An ideal gift to a vet or animal owner is a ribbon-wrapped bouquet of clubmoss sprigs which they can hang in their home, animal-treatment room, or wherever the animal lives.

Cowslips

Primula veris. Attribution: Venus (Culpeper)
Cowslips are small plants with hanging yellow bell-shaped flowers. In Somerset, people carry cowslips when they are seeking treasure or trying to penetrate the haunts of fairies, because doing so makes these places apparent. However, for it to work, they say, you must carry the right number and go forth at the right time.[116]

∞ **Cowslips for seeing fairies.** Carry cowslips with you when going out into nature for the purpose of finding fairies. We do not know what old Somerset folk consider to be 'the right time', but it is generally understood that one seeks them at night, either on the full moon or on a night when the veil between the worlds is thin, such as May Eve. Cowslips blossom in April and May, so these are a flower you can carry with you on such a night. The places of the fairies will be apparent to you if everything has been done properly and you are sufficiently attuned. We suggest wearing green clothes for the outing, as this is the colour of the fey folk, and wearing the colour is a sign that you come in a spirit of kinship with them. Always bring with you something to offer the fairies; it is said they like milk, cream and alcoholic drinks.

∞ **Cowslips for finding treasure.** To use cowslips to find treasure, follow the instructions above for using them to see fairies. In this instance, however, attune your senses to perceiving treasures in the landscape, rather than the abodes of the fairies. We suggest carrying with you a small piece of the kind of treasure that you seek, on the principle of like attracts like.

Crocus flowers (saffron)

Crocus sativus. Attribution: Sun (Culpeper, saffron crocus)
Stamens of the crocus flower produce the valuable saffron powder widely used in ancient magic and worship. The Phoenicians honoured the goddess Ashtoreth (Ishtar/Astarte) by baking and eating moon-shaped cakes which contained saffron; this goddess has the power to bestow power and fertility. In ancient Egypt, saffron was considered sacred to the sun. Known as the 'blood of Thoth', it was burnt in rituals to Thoth.[117] In Europe, it has appeared in folk magic since the Middle Ages—but one must be aware that juniper was also sometimes called saffron in Britain. Numerous regional customs prescribe crocus saffron to make a person joyful and prone to laughter, most commonly through a tea or as a food seasoning.[118] It is also used in love spells, as it has the power to make people feel romantic.[119]

∞ **Saffron for erotic love.** Include saffron in love potions and sex spells. A tiny pinch of saffron is easily added to a love drink or love tea, which is made from a selection of love-inducing herbs and spices; the full list can be found at the beginning of the book.

∞ **Saffron for strength.** Saffron is a magnificent strengthening herb, particularly when eaten while honouring the goddess Ashtoreth/Isthar/Astarte. Bake moon-shaped cakes and flavour them with a tiny pinch of saffron.

∞ **Saffron for becoming a great magician.** Thoth is the patron of learned magicians, and saffron is sacred to him. Burn a little saffron on charcoal as an incense while mentally honouring Thoth.

∞ **Saffron for joy.** Use saffron in spells for happiness, as it has the magical ability to produce happiness and laughter.

A nice way to do this is to make small cakes seasoned with saffron. Other joy-inducing herbs can be added to the mix, depending on what you like and what you have available to you.

∞ **Saffron for love.** Include it in love spells, particularly in cases where happiness and joy are called for. It is also a good ingredient for love spells in which the object of affection is a magician or a scholar, because saffron is sacred to the god Thoth, who is patron of both pursuits.

Cyclamen
Also known as sow bread
Genus *Cyclamen*. Attribution: Mars (Culpeper)
Today, most people encounter the cyclamen flower as a potted plant, one that is commonly given as gift. It is distinctive for its delicate, unusually shaped flowers, which sit atop fragile stalks. English lore says that cyclamen has the power to make someone love you.[120] The Greeks used it for protection: Pliny wrote that every home should grow it, as no evil magic can take effect in a place where it grows.[121] An old poem relates how a woman protected a man in her care from psychic attack using this flower:

> St John's Wort and fresh Cyclamen she in her chamber kept
> From the power of evil angels to guard him while he slept.[122]

∞ **Cyclamen for protection.** Keep a potted cyclamen in your house for protection. It is a lovely gift to a friend who has moved to a new home, or who is going through a difficult time. As it is not unusual to give a friend or neighbour a potted cyclamen, you can give it without stating its magical powers to the recipient. Only you need know that it will grant them good powers; it is a simple way to give a blessing to a non-magically inclined person you are fond of.

∞ **Cyclamen for love.** Use cyclamen in love spells which involve making a specific person fall in love with you. We recommend using a few flower petals in the mixture.

Cypress

Cupressus sempervirens. Attribution: Saturn (Culpeper and Lilly)

This evergreen, which grows all across the Mediterranean region as well as further north across Europe, has been considered sacred since ancient times. Since the earliest records, it has been considered a tree of sorrow, mourning and grief. It is often found in cemeteries and graveyards.[123] In Cambridgeshire, people believe that the spirits of the dead shelter under its branches in graveyards and so avoid them.[124] But for all its sad associations, it is a plant of good powers: it has long been used in exorcisms. The medieval mystic-physician Hildegard of Bingen used it in this way. Here is her method.

Hildegard's Cypress-and-Water Exorcism

When someone has been ensnared by a diabolic or magical force, this is how to proceed. Take a piece of wood from the heart of a cypress tree and drill a hole in it. Then you must fill a jug with water from a living spring, pour this water through the drilled hole, and collect it once more. Meanwhile speak the following incantation. 'I pour you, o water, through this hole; so that the strength which characterises you will flow into the person's lost soul; so that all that is bad and hostile within him [or her] will be destroyed. And that he [or she] will be placed back on the path which God set him.'[125]

Better than cure is prevention, of course, and Hildegard suggests that people wear a twig of cypress to prevent evil forces reaching them in the first place. Indeed, it is a common practice to carry a little bit of cypress for protection.[126]

Cypress is also used in spells. Folklore says that if you want to cast a spell upon an enemy, follow them so you can identify their footprints, then place cypress branches or twigs over the tracks: if you do this, you will have control over them.[127]

∽   **Cypress for exorcism.** In the case of a poltergeist or unwanted supernatural activity in a place, use cypress in your clearing rite. We suggest using the cypress as a water sprinkler, bearing in mind that it is a common practice in spirit-banishing to sprinkle the home with saltwater or puri-fied water. Cypress needles or twigs can be burned as an incense so that cypress essence fills the air.

✿   **Cypress for protection.** Carry a sprig of cypress or keep it in your pocket. We suggest carrying this particular plant when you are bereaved or are dealing with matters of death.

✿   **Cypress for control.** Place the cypress in the footprint of the person you wish to control. We urge caution and restraint in all situations in which you are tempted to override another person's will; it is advisable to first undertake a period of self-reflection, to assess your ethics and personal responsibility.

Daffodil
Also known as narcissus, asphodel
Genus *Amaryllidaceae*. Attribution: Mercury (Culpeper), Venus (Lilly), Saturn (Albertus Magnus)
Much English folklore says the daffodil brings ill fortune if it comes into your home.[128] Albertus Magnus' Book of Secrets, however, says it is good to have it inside, because 'it suf-fereth not a devil in the house'.[129] The same work, popular in France right up into the twentieth century, says that to cure demonic possession or madness, you should carry a daffodil wrapped in a clean napkin.[130]

✿   **Daffodil for mental wellbeing.** Place daffodils in a vase wrapped with a clean white piece of cloth for mental wellbeing. We suggest that when using daffodils you do this outside your home; for example, at your workplace or in an outdoor environment. However, if you are unconcerned by the old English taboo, you can certainly have them in the place you live.

Daisy
Also known as English daisy, common daisy
Genus *Bellis*. Attribution: Venus (Culpeper)
The daisy is one of the most common English flowers, grow-ing both in gardens and in the wild. According to Somerset

lore, the daisy is a woman's flower. A daisy chain is made and put on a child to give it protection in Somerset, and also in Devon, where the daisy chain specifically keeps the child from being kidnapped by fairies.[131] Ox-eye daisies (their old name is moon daisies) are used in an old Somerset charm to bring back an unfaithful lover.[132]

∽ **Daisy for a child blessing.** Make a daisy chain for a child and place it either around their neck or on their head as a crown. A summer birthday is an ideal time for this, and it can easily be done at a celebratory picnic or outdoor party. It is also a nice thing to do if you have moved house and have come to a new neighbourhood, as it is a way to connect to the new locality, its spirit and its plant realm.

∽ **Daisy to bring back a lover.** Include ox-eye daisies in your spell and have them in your house.

Dill

Anethum graveolens. Attribution: Mercury (Culpeper)

Nowadays, we mainly know dill as a cooking herb, but it is a potent magical plant; it is called 'the magician's herb' in some places.[133] Dill has great power to protect people from bad magic and malevolent spirits; as the old saying goes, 'The vervain and the dill, That hindreth witches of their will.'[134] German folklore says dill above the door will keep the envious out of your home.[135] In some regions, dill is used in sex magic, because it has the power to arouse passion.[136]

∽ **Dill against evil envy.** Put dill at the edges of the spaces or objects which are the object of envy.

∽ **Dill for passion.** Use dill in spells when you want to make your partner passionate about you once again. Use it also when you need a boost of your own passion for your partner. It is also good for making a platonic friend feel attracted to you.

∽ **Dill for protection.** Use dill to protect against misfortune or evil magic.

Elder

Sambucus nigra. Attribution: Venus (Culpeper), Mercury (Lilly)

The elder is one of the most magically potent trees of all. Though most English people know it only through elderflower cordial, this delicately flowering tree is hardly benign. It has a dark and haunting reality, and all across Europe people have long known it is the home of dangerous supernatural entities. The biggest taboo involves cutting it in any way.

As for who the elder spirit is, beliefs vary. Some regions hold that it is witches and elves who live in the elder and that they bury their children under its roots; the dead children of the witches revive as bees, butterflies or caterpillars on the elder branches.[137] Others say that it is fairies who live there. Follow the instructions below to have a conference with a fairy.

The Magram Fairy Spell

Find an elder tree; stroll underneath it at midday; while underneath it say three times, 'Magram Magrano'; a fair woman will appear, from whom you may ask a wish, which she will grant; a yellow flower will spring up, which you are to pick: when you hold this flower you will want nothing.[138]

Danish lore says the elder is inhabited by an elder mother, so they do not use elder for furniture. To cut it for firewood, in Lower Saxony, you say, 'Lady Elder, Give me some of thy wood, Then I will give thee some of mine, When it grows in the forest.'[139]

The lady of the elder is often unspecified, but in Denmark she is understood to be the goddess Holda; elder was used in rites to Holda on the Venusberg.[140] Holda is involved in a special spell, which is here quoted verbatim from Skinner:

Holda's Twelfth Night Elder Spell

On the night of January 6 you may cut a branch from the elder tree, first having asked permission, and spat thrice if no answer comes from the wood. With the branch you will mark a magic circle in a lonely field, stand at the centre, surrounded with such kinds of bloom and berry as you have saved from St John's night, and, so prepared, you will demand of the devil, then abroad, some of his precious fern-seed that gives to you the strength of thirty men. Though the evil one is foot-free on that night, he is still under the spell of the good Hulda, and when a wand of her wood is directed against him he must obey, and the fern-seed will be brought by a shadowy somebody, folded in a chalice cloth.[141]

In Britain and Scotland, the inhabitant of the elder tree is usually unspecified, but it clearly is a spirit, and gaining its permission is essential. This is a widespread taboo, so just one specific example is given by the Victorian folklorist who relates the following collected lore: you must say, 'Elder, Elder, may I cut thy branches? If there is no sign of disapproval, you can cut the tree after you have spit three times.[142] In Scotland, many people will not burn elder wood at all, because to do so would 'raise the Devil' or cause a death in the family.[143] That said, in parts of Scotland, on the eve of May Day it was customary to gather elderflowers and elder branches (presumably, having asked permission) and to put them over doors and windows to keep out bad magic.[144] In parts of England, St John's Eve (24th of June) was the day on which to collect the elder which would give you protection.[145]

∞　**Elder to see fairies.** Go to an elder grove and wait to see the fairies. We recommend making it into a small pilgrimage: pack a picnic, take a cushion to sit upon, or even a sleeping bag in order to stay overnight. Be sure to respectfully greet the tree when you arrive and give it an offering. If you do this expedition in winter, we suggest organising it for the night of 6 January. If in summer, we recommend Midsummer's Day at noon.

∞　**Elder to get a wish.** Perform the Magram Spell above

∞　**Elder for physical prowess.** Perform the fern-seed spell above with an elderwood wand.

∞　**Elder against evil forces.** Make a wand of elder wood, having carefully asked the elder tree for permission before cutting it. It is a good idea to use an elder branch which has fallen naturally from the tree so you do not cut the tree at all.

∞ **Elder for protection.** On May Day or at midsummer, collect elderflowers and put them on your door lintel and windows.

Elm

Genus *Ulnus*. Attribution: Saturn (Culpeper)
In Europe, the elm is known to have the power to ward off demons and spirits, and so is widely used in magic. Some English sorcerers make their magic wands from wych elm wood; it is considered the most magically potent variety of elm. The most common ways of employing the power of the elm tree is to cut sticks and place them around the place to be protected, or to carry twigs of elm in one's pocket.[146]

∞ **Elm for protection of a space.** Find a local elm tree and collect sticks from fallen branches; elms have had their numbers vastly reduced due to disease, so do not cut any elm tree in any way. We recommend asking the blessing of the elm tree before taking the wood. Place them around the space you want to be protected.

∞ **Elm for personal protection.** Carry elm twigs in your pocket or in your clothing.

∞ **Elm for magical tools.** Craft your magic wand from wych elm wood.

Fennel

Foeniculum vulgare. Attribution: Mercury (Culpeper)
Aromatic fennel is a staple of herbalism and in cooking. Going back as far as the early Middle Ages, it has been considered a very powerful magical plant, partly because of its strong scent.

Over many parts of Europe, and in England's county of Somerset, people hang bunches of it over their doors on Midsummer's Eve to ward off evil spirits.[147] Some people even stuff pinches of it into keyholes so that magicians can't enter. In France's Béarn region, it is done with this rhyme:

> If a wizard tries to enter
> Through this hole today,
> Have a good sniff, Fennel!
> He will get a fright
> And dare not enter.[148]

∞ **Fennel for protection.** Put fennel around your home, your workspace or any other place where you feel that you need protection. It is especially good to use fennel that has been gathered on Midsummer's Day, or to put it out on Midsummer's Day. You can put it into the keyholes while reciting the rhyme above, if you wish.

Fern, bracken

Pteridium aquilinum. Attribution: Mercury (Culpeper)

Fern is one of the most lore-rich plants in Europe. An old Catholic church calendar's note for 22–3 June reads, 'Fern is in great estimation with the vulgar, on account of its seed.'[149] The fern is an uncanny plant, odd—on account of its apparent lack of flowers and for its strange tiny seeds. Lyte writes, 'this kinde of Ferne beareth neither flowers nor sede, except we shall take for sede the black spots growing on the back sides of the leaves, the which some to gather, thinking to worke wonders'.[150]

Wonders indeed. Fern seeds scattered on the ground on St John's Eve will reveal any buried treasure by glowing blue; you will see them in 'a dim blue light, as if the earth were glass'.[151] Fern seeds, say others, have the power to confer invisibility: Ben Jonson's *New Inn* has the line 'I had no medicine, Sir, to go invisible, no Fern seed in my pocket.'

There are rituals for gathering the seeds. John Aubrey's method is a technique related to him by someone who swore they actually did it. Late on St John's Eve, go out alone to the fern. Crouch over it, lay a white napkin underneath the fern's branches and wait for the seed to fall on to it. When the seed falls, the elves will whisk you about the ears.

Aubrey's friend's method is not the only one. One Victorian folklore writer relates another way. On Christmas, just before midnight, go with a chalice cloth to a crossroads which has recently had a corpse taken through it. Stand in silence; supernatural beings will come to you, cuff your ears or knock off your hat and make mysterious noises to try to make you speak. Resist them and stay silent, then walk forward, still in silence. You will see snakes running over the frozen earth; they will lead you to the fern, which you will see with its seed, glowing and sparkling. Catch the seed in the cloth before the sun rises.[152] Many other similar fern-collecting instructions have been gathered from around the British Isles.[153]

A third method is this: the seed-hunter must avoid going to church during Epiphany and in this time concentrate on contemplating Satan; when Epiphany is over, he can collect the seed, which is under the keeping of Satan. But is it really Satan? One seventeenth-century interviewee was insistent that it was rather the King of the Fairies who ruled the seed.[154] The Cornish, too, hold that it is the fairies who live in fern beds: 'All ferns are haunts of the fairies, who in Cornwall are the spirits of such as died in paganism, before the coming of Christ, and are punished for lacking the true faith by the shortening of stature and the strange life of the woods.'[155]

∽ **Collect fern seed.** Read the methods which have been used in the past, noting dates, times and actions. Devise your own, based upon what is practical for you, having found a fern bank nearby. Our only additional suggestion is to take a small offering for the spirits.

∽ **Visit fern patches to see fairies.** The best time to find fairies in fern beds is just before midnight, and it is recommended to try to do this just after Epiphany (the season running from 6 January until the last Sunday before Ash Wednesday). You should have avoided going to church throughout Epiphany. Alternatively, you can try on Christmas night itself. We recommend taking a gift for the fairies; they are said to like milk, cream and alcoholic spirits, but use your initiative.

Feverfew

Tanacetum parthenium. Attribution: Venus (Culpeper), Jupiter (Lilly)
Feverfew is found in verges and on waste ground: it's a hardy plant whose flowers look like tiny daisies growing in bunches.

It is mainly used medicinally rather than magically, but one old piece of lore asserts that feverfew will help a person feel better when they are pensive, sad and don't want to talk to anyone.[156]

  ∿ **Feverfew against melancholic non-communication.** Use this herb in a magical tea to help a person who is silently miserable feel better and more communicative. If you are able, serve the tea in a cup which is either orange or multi-coloured; doing so infuses the drink with even more mercurial, communicative energy.

Fig tree

Genus *Ficus.* Attribution: Jupiter (Culpeper), Venus (Lilly)

In Christianity, some think it was the fig that was the original tree of knowledge, rather than the apple.[157] In Italy, a gesture of insult is the mano in fica; the fingers folded into the hand make it resemble a fig, which is a euphemism for the vulva. So, the fig has connotations of women's sexuality, and women's vulvas in particular. In some folklore, the fig has the power to instil calm: if a raging bull is tied to a fig tree, he will become 'tame and gentle'.[158]

The fig tree is a portal to otherworldly beings—just as the elm and the walnut are, in some areas of Europe. Like the walnut tree, in Italy the fig is a tree of psychic misfortune, or—at best—psychic danger.[159] Skinner relates that people are warned about falling asleep under a fig tree. If you do so, there is a chance that you will be awakened by a supernatural figure, a woman who looks to be the ghost of a nun. She will offer you a knife, holding it out to you. If you reach to take it by the blade, she will pierce you in the heart. But if you grasp it by the handle, she will give you good fortune.[160]

  ∿ **Fig in spells for women's sexual pleasure or sexuality.** In your spell, use the fig to represent the vulva. Ideally, pluck the fruit from a tree near you, if this is possible. Alternatively, you could buy a fresh fig when in season, and some shops sell jars of figs in syrup. Either of these is preferable to using dried figs, for obvious reasons. If you are seeking to increase passionate, driven sex, perform the spell on a Tuesday, but if you are seeking to create relaxed, languorous eroticism, do it on a Friday.

∽ **Fig to dissipate anger.** Use fig, or go to a fig tree, to calm someone from a rage. If you are aiming to bring down your own temper, we recommend going to sit under a fig tree, making it a small pilgrimage. If you need to calm another person or an animal, lead them to the tree and settle them under its branches. We suggest you take an offering to the tree, then settle down seated under its branches, perhaps leaning your back against its trunk.

∽ **Fig to meet supernatural spirits.** To meet the mysterious grey lady of the fig tree, prepare an overnight stay under a tree, making sure you can do so safely. Choose a clear night without rain in one of the warmer months of the year. It's best to do it on a full moon. Take a warm sleeping bag to sleep in the open air or, if that does not appeal, pitch a small tent under the tree. Before you close your eyes for the night, drink some herbal tea from a flask: a tisane of one of the herbs which has the power of helping you dream true. Remember, when the woman who appears offers you the knife, you should take it by the handle, not the blade.

Fir

Genus *Abies*. Attribution: Mars/Jupiter (Culpeper)[161]
Fir was sacred to pagans in pre-Christian France: when St Martin arrived and destroyed the pagan temples, the local people refused to let him destroy the fir trees.[162] In the northern countries, the fir is the king of the forest and home to a living spirit, so people will not cut it. In Russia, when a giant fir is knocked down by a storm the locals will not sell the wood but instead insist upon giving it to the church. In German regions, it is exceptionally important; in the Harz region, there is a custom of dancing around a fir tree to win favours from the resident tree spirit.[163]

To stop nightmares, says one old charm, put a branch of fir on your bed.[164] In fact, people used fir to keep away supernatural beings who steal things: it is an old custom to put a branch of fir at the door of a store-room or storehouse, so that the goods inside cannot be taken by a supernatural thief. A sprig of fir is also employed to keep away the spirits that torment people's sleep.[165]

∽ **Fir for curing nightmares.** Find a fir growing locally and cut a sprig, first asking the blessing of the tree. Tie it to your bed. We recommend doing this on a Monday, the day of sleep and dreams (the moon's day), and tying the sprig to your bed using a red thread, which is the colour of the tree's energy (Mars). If your bed does not have a frame on to which you can tie the fir twig, you can put it under your pillow to achieve the same effect.

∽ **Fir to prevent theft.** Put fir branches or fir needles around your store-room or storehouse to keep it safe from supernatural beings who might want to spirit away your precious belongings. Christina's tip: similarly, use it to deter human burglars.

∽ **To get a wish.** Dance around a fir tree asking the tree spirit to grant you your favour. We recommend that you make an offering to the tree, as it is courteous to do so when asking a favour.

Forget-me-not
Also known as mouse-ear, scorpion grass
Myosotis sylvatica. Attribution: Moon (Culpeper)
In Somerset, these pretty little blue wildflowers should be carried when you go out seeking treasure or to find the haunts of fairies. If you do take a little bouquet of forget-me-nots, you will find what you seek. However, the tradition says you must use the right number of flowers, and do so at the right time.[166]

∽ **Forget-me-nots for wealth.** Carry forget-me-nots into meetings where you are negotiating for more pay or which are about financial deals; also, take some with you as you set out on wealth-accruing missions.

∽ **Forget-me-nots to find the dwellings of spirits and fairies.** Carry forget-me-nots with you on outings to encounter

60

fairies, We recommend making such excursions at night, ideally around midnight on a full moon, and that you visit a local wooded area, in particular seeking out a bower of the sorts of trees in which fairies are said to live and congregate (elm, walnut, and so on).

Fuller's teasel

Also known as wild teasel, fuller's thistle, manured teasel
Dipsacus fullonum, syn. *Dipsacus sylvestris.* Attribution: Venus (Culpeper)
This thistle-like flowering plant was used in olden times by fabric fullers to 'tease' wool and flax cloth as part of its preparation. It is not much used in folk magic. One magical use in Switzerland is for protection against gunshot or stabbing.

Swiss Bulletproofing and Stab-proofing Charm
Prepare a piece of black cloth that is brand new. Find some local plants of fuller's teasel. Then go back on the eve of the day of St John the Baptist (Midsummer's Eve), after the sun has set fully and it is completely dark, bringing the cloth with you. Find three plants which no longer have their tips. Harvest them as you say these words: 'I am taking you for all the virtue you that you may hold.' Or these:

> I take you that you may have the strength,
> by the virtue given to you by God,
> to defend me against swords and bullets,
> and against all kinds of firearms.
> In the name of the Father, the Son, and the Holy Ghost.

Wrap them in the cloth. Carry this bundle with you. If you do so, such is the virtue of this root that 'you shall never be wounded by any arm, whether you find yourself in battle or elsewhere'.[167]

∞   **Fuller's teasel for bulletproofing.** Perform the ritual outlined above.

Garlic

Genus *allium*. Attribution: Mars (Culpeper, Lilly)

Garlic was sacred to Hecate and was placed at crossroads in her honour.[168] All across Europe, it is employed against the evil eye or witchcraft; wearing a necklace of garlic is a classic method. In Bulgaria, it is customary to hang it over the door to keep out the bad luck caused by jealous or envious ill-wishing people. Alternatively, you can rub your pots, kettles and pans with garlic for the same effect.[169]

∞ **Garlic for protection against jealousy and envy.** Rub garlic on those of your possessions that people covet, or for which they resent you. We advise doing this on a Tuesday, the day of the fiery energy we call Mars. It is probably best to use garlic as a protection when the object and space are related to cooking, the kitchen or a restaurant, since its odour is quite pungent.

∞ **Garlic for personal protection.** Wear a garlic necklace. Alternatively, include a bit of dried garlic, powdered, in potions containing a mixture of herbs.

Greater stitchwort

Also known as cuckoo-flower, ladies' smock

Stellaria lolostea. Attribution: Moon (Culpeper)

This grass-like meadow wildflower, with its small, white, star-shaped flowers, is common across Britain and Ireland. It features in plant magic only rarely. In Somerset, it is called 'pixies', and there it is believed that if you go out to fetch greater stitchwort, you are likely to be pixie-led.[170] That is to say, the fairies or pixies will come and take you away to their realm.

∞ **Greater stitchwort to enter the fairy realm.** Go out into a remote area, away from other people, and gather this flower. We recommend doing this on the day of the full moon, or on May Eve or at midsummer. It should always be done alone, and you should take gifts for the fey folk: milk, cream and whiskey are traditional.

Ground ivy

Also known as alehoof
Glechoma hederacea. Attribution: Venus (Culpeper)
This is a low, creeping plant with kidney-shaped leaves and tiny purple flowers. If you wear some ground ivy, you will be able to perceive whom of those around you are witches and who are simply normal folk.[171]

∽ **Ground ivy to see people's hidden dark sides.** If you wish to see other aspects of people around you, for good or for ill, you can make use of this old charm, which is to wear a sprig of this herb. In its old form, it says you will see witches, which in those days meant ordinary people who had a hidden, secret side to their lives in which they caused harm to others. Now, as in the past, there are people who have hidden sides to their personalities, who are hypocritical and lead double lives in which they secretly cause hurt. These people are often charming, and they often 'groom' their unsuspecting acquaintances. To see through this, the ground ivy's powers can be called upon. It is best to do this at midnight on the night of the full moon. Prepare yourself and the space for the occasion. If there is a person or people you are concerned about, set out a photo or picture of them, nail clippings, hair or any other symbolic representation; surround these items with a circle of salt. When midnight strikes, ask the assistance of the ground-ivy plant, then burn some dried herbs as an incense on some charcoals, at the same time charging up a small wrap of it. Sprinkle the items in the salt circle with saltwater. When you have finished, put all the items outside, or burn them, except the wrap of ground ivy, which you should wear on you. In the coming days, as you meet people in your daily life, you will be shown whether or not they are evil-doers.

Hawthorn

Also known as whitethorn, may tree
Crataegus monogyna. Attribution: Mars (Culpeper)
Hawthorn is one of the top magical plants of the British Isles. It is a thorny bush which sometimes grows into a large tree and is common across the British Isles. Its distinguishing features are the fact that it blossoms around May Day and that

its white blossom contains chemical compounds that make it smell of death and sex. Two species of hawthorn are found in England: the common hawthorn, which is found everywhere (*Crataegus monogyna*), and the midland hawthorn (*Crataegus laevigata*) of central/ south-east England. The latter is the species which famously smells of putrid flesh, as it contains trimethylamine, a chemical emitted from dying bodies.[172] In ancient Greece, it was the tree that was sacred to Cardea, a death goddess. Cardea wove spells with her hawthorn wand and was an enemy of children. Hawthorn blossom taken into the house was sure to be followed by Cardea, so it was prohibited to bring hawthorn in.[173] This prohibition remained almost universal across Europe—it is certainly the normal taboo in the British Isles up to the present day.

The lore on hawthorn is often seasonal to May Day. One must wear, bear and/or decorate with hawthorn on May Day; this is one of the oldest and most widespread customs across the British Isles. To quote just one example of hundreds, it is said, in Somerset, 'You must have whitethorn in your May tutti.'[174]

The hawthorn tree is a common place for fairies to make their home. It is a belief across Britain that a hawthorn bush on its own in a field or an open area is the home of the local fairies and must be respected.[175] In many locations, it is customary for people to dance around such a lone hawthorn tree at May Day.[176] It is widely known that in a garden or anywhere outdoors, if you find an oak tree, ash tree and hawthorn tree growing in such a way as to form a natural triangle in the landscape, then within that triangle you can see fairies; it is suggested this was the code embedded in the Kipling poem 'Oak and Ash and Thorn'.

For all that it is a plant associated with fairies and the supernatural, hawthorn is also a tree for protection, even apart from around May Day. A sprig of hawthorn was a common good-luck charm to go above a baby's cradle in ancient Rome, and even into the twentieth century it was a French custom to do the same.[177]

∞　**Hawthorn to see fairies.** Go to visit a lone hawthorn tree; try to do so on May Day or the night before, May

Eve (Beltane, i.e. the night of 30 April); if you want to do this sooner, we advise going out on a special day such as Midsummer's Day, Hallowe'en or on a night of the full moon. The fairies are best approached with offerings, and they are known to like cream, milk and whiskey. We advise going out at midnight, the time when the barrier between the supernatural realms and the mortal realms is most penetrable.

 ⧼ **Hawthorn for good fortune.** Wear hawthorn on May Day, and decorate your door lintels with it. We recommend tying your garlands and adornments with thread of red and green, the colours of passion and love.

 ⧼ **Hawthorn for a baby blessing.** Include hawthorn in a bag or bouquet to be hung up near a baby's cradle. As with all baby-blessing charms which contain herbs, specify to the parents that they need to keep it far enough away from the baby that there is no chance the baby will get hold of it to nibble on its contents.

Hazel

Genus *Corylus*. Attribution: Mercury (Culpeper), Jupiter (Lilly)
Hazel is a tree of magic going back to the ancient world; since that time, it continues to be the most prescribed wood for making magical wands.[178] In one version of the biblical legend, Aaron's rod was made of hazel. And in the ancient world, 'the hazel is the caduceus of Mercury, which roused in all who were touched by it love of kin, country, and the gods'.[179] Circe's wand was allegedly made of hazel, a wand she used to turn her lovers into swine. In Ireland, it was said to be 'a wand of hazel with which St Patrick drove the Irish snakes into the sea'. Medieval magicians' wands were made of hazel, and they use them when summoning angels and demons. An early modern English writer related this working involving hazel wands, the aim of which is to 'get a fayrie:'

Suffolk Fayrie Spell

First, get a broad square christall or Venice glasse, in length and bredth three inches. Then lay that glasse or christall in the blood of a white henne, three Wednesdayes or three Fridayes. Then take it out and wash it with holy aqua [water] and fumigate it. Then take three hazel sticks, or wands, of an [one] year growth; pill [peel] the fayre and white; and make the soe longe as you can write the spiritt's name, or fayrie's name, which you call three times on evry stick being made flatt on one side. Then bury them under some hill, whereat you suppose fayries haunt, the Wednesday before you call her: and the Friday following take them uppe and call her at eight, or three, or ten of the clocke, which be good planets and hours for that turne; but when you call be in cleane life and turn thy face towards the East, and when you have her bind her in that stone and glasse.[180]

Hazel wands were employed by people of all stripes, all across Europe, from farmer to cunning man; the hazel wand is used for 'securing crops, warding off lightning, curing fever, and driving devils out of cattle'.[181] Old folklore of England says to draw a circle around oneself using a hazel wand to protect yourself from supernatural attack by 'evil spirits and evil hands', fairies, and other ghostly creatures; the hazel is only effective if it is cut after May Day, when it gains its power.[182] In Germany, hazel wood was employed specifically.[183] There it was used for making the dowsing rods in the mining areas of England, where dowsers would search for mineral seams.[184] Sailors at sea would wear a sprig or crown of it to prevent death by shipwreck.[185]

The nuts of the hazel have magical powers, too. In Ireland, they are understood to confer wisdom, as attested across old Irish myths: 'the hazels of wisdom' appear in several points in the sagas, together with the salmon, a fish that eats the nuts and is a patron of wisdom. And, in more recent folk belief, hazelnuts are said to confer invisibility.[186]

∞   **Hazel for magical tools.** Use hazel when making a magic wand, to follow in this long and esteemed lineage. Some people say you must cut it after May Day, and we suggest following this guideline. The traditional time to do this is on the day and hour of Mercury, which is easily established: it is every Wednesday morning at sunrise. Magical custom says that, ideally, you should cut your wand in a single stroke. If you wish to do this, you will need to choose a branch that is no thicker than a finger, and use large secateurs, both of which are most easily achieved if you plan the cutting expedition in advance.

∞ **Hazel for invisibility.** Use hazelnuts for an invisibility spell. We suggest that the 'charged up' nuts are placed in a pouch or wrap in which you can carry them in a pocket or a bag. The wrap should be orange, the colour of Mercurial energy, which is trickster energy.

∞ **Hazel for gaining wisdom.** Use hazelnuts in your working. We suggest that you be sure to eat them at the end of the spell. Further research into Irish lore on hazelnuts will assist you in creating a special ceremony full of symbolic meaning, out of which you will gain insight and maturity—the components of wisdom.

∞ **Hazel for protection at sea.** Put some hazel on the boat, or carry some on you when you are sailing or travelling at sea. Alternatively, put a little hazel in your safety jacket or your sun hat.

∞ **Hazel for protection against dangerous supernatural forces.** Cut a hazel wand after May Day, and use it whenever you feel in danger, at which time you should use it to draw a circle around yourself.

Henbane

Genus *Hyoscyamus*. Attribution: Saturn (Culpeper), Jupiter (Albertus Magnus)

Henbane is one of the herbs most deeply associated with witches and witches' potions and dark spells.[187] As a drug, it is fatal, so it must never be eaten or drunk. It was known in the Middle Ages: fourteenth-century author Bartholomeus wrote, 'this herb is called insana wood, for the use thereof is perilous; for if it be eate or dranke, it breedeth woodenes, or slow liknes of slepe; therefore the herb is commonly called Morilindi, for it taketh away wytte and reason'.[188] It was one of the ingredients of the legendary witches' ointment. Culpeper unsurprisingly attributed Saturnian energy to the plant, criticising the author of the Book of Secrets of Albertus Magnus, which had given it to Jupiter. It is a plant traditionally gathered at midsummer, when its power is believed to be at its strongest.[189]

Henbane features in numerous magical workings. Agrippa's work on plants (*De vegetalibus*) says that if a magician wants to cast a spell on a person, they should start by drawing a sketch of the victim, using henbane juice for ink. The image drawn, combined with the power of the herb, serves to start the process of the enchantment.[190] It can cause bitter enmity between lovers and spouses: one old German curse is to place henbane seeds between two members of a couple, because it would be sure to cause them 'to live in hatred'.[191]

Henbane is also effective in love spells and is widely used for that purpose, going back to the sixteenth century and possibly before.[192] *The Book of Secrets* says that you should carry a sprig of it on yourself to enjoy a high sex drive and be attractive to others: 'It is profitable to them that would do often the act of generation; and to them that desire to be loved of women, it is good they bear it with them, for it maketh the bearers pleasant and delectable.'[193] Henbane's power of creating attraction is evident in this old German spell: if a shopkeeper sprinkles henbane seeds in their shop window or in front of their products, customers always flock to the items and rush to buy them.[194]

WARNING: Henbane is fatal if consumed. Do not swallow even a tiny amount. Do not burn it, as you can die from breathing the fumes.

Herb bennet

Also known as wood avens, avens, clovewort, herb bonet
Genus *Geum urbanum*. Attribution: Jupiter (Culpeper)
This plant, with its tiny yellow flowers, grows wild at woodland edges and near hedgerows. Its name is derived from the Latin word benedictus, meaning 'blessed', and herb bennet is used as protection against evil. In some places, the root is used; it smells like cloves when it is dug up; it is then worn around the

neck so the wearer will never be attacked by wild beasts.[195] In Somerset, it is grown near the house to prevent the devil getting in; folklore says that where herb bennet is, the evil one cannot approach.[196]

✐ **Herb bennet for protection against attack by animals, gang violence or muggers.** Use herb bennet in protection spells or put it on your person or at the borders of your home. We recommend finding a plant near your home, then digging it up on a Thursday (the day of Jupiter) to get the aromatic root. Wrap the root in purple string (or fabric) and wear it around your neck. This is an amulet you might want to make for a friend who is around animals who are troubled: a rescue-shelter worker or mail deliverer. After all, it is well known that some dogs are aggressive towards postal workers, making their job stressful. The amulet is effective against humans who are violently out of control and are in attack mode, be it teens in a gang, angry drunks on the street or muggers.

✐ **Herb bennet for home protection.** Plant it near your house, ideally near the front door or the place where you are most concerned about unwelcome people being.

Herb-paris
Also known as herb truelove, one-berry
Paris quadrifolia. Attribution: Venus (Culpeper)
This shade-loving plant is distinctive for its shape: four wide leaves set in a cross. Joined at the centre, they create a looped love-knot with a single black berry in the centre. Herb-paris used to be common in the West of England. In sixteenth-century Italy, its berries were used to restore the sanity of people who had 'lost their minds through bewitchment', as reported by a contemporary physician, Mattioli.[197] The same remedy was used in seventeenth-century Germany.[198] The berry is poisonous, so do not eat it.

✐ **Herb-paris for spiritual equilibrium.** Use herb-paris in spells to relieve supernaturally induced instability. We suggest using a living plant growing in a pot and making it the centrepiece of a meditation in which you contemplate its equal-armed leaves, which are an outward expression of its equanimity, its balance and its stability. The four classic elements—earth, air, fire and water—were qualities in the world and in each person; when they are in balance, harmony is the result. To do such a meditation, we suggest using a compass and aligning the four leaves with the four points of the compass. Place candles around your plant as follows: green for north, yellow for east, red for south, blue for west. Turn the lights down and have gentle music playing in the background. Attune to the plant as a living being who is benevolent, gentle and calm, then do a moving meditation, circling the plant as you intuitively wish to. At the end of the working, thank the plant. Then keep it in your home, tending it lovingly.

Herb robert

Also known as red robin, death-come-quickly
Geranium robertianum. Attribution: Venus (Culpeper)
This low-growing plant, with its small pink flowers, is a widespread weed which grows amidst the grass of lawns. In Somerset, it is believed that if you pick it, the fairies will come and get you: 'If 'ee pick'n, someone'll take 'ee.'[199]

∞   **Herb robert to enter fairy realms.** Go out and pick herb robert in a remote area, on your own. The fairies are easiest to see and meet on certain nights of the year, so we recommend doing this endeavour on one of these: May Eve, Midsummer's Eve, or Hallowe'en. If you do not want to wait until one of these dates, the next best option is to go out on a full moon, at midnight. Plan where you are going in advance: on a map or in person, find the nearest wooded area which is rarely visited by people, looking particularly for an overgrown sheltered grove within it. Alternatively, seek in the open lands a single-standing hawthorn tree. These are likely dwelling places. On the night, we advise taking gifts for the fairies, noting that they are said to like alcoholic drinks, milk and cream.

Holly

Genus *Ilex*. Attribution: Saturn (Culpeper)

Holly is one of the winter seasonal evergreens used to decorate the home during the twelve days of Christmas, a custom which is probably a survival of the Roman use of holly at Saturnalia. In Christian lore, the holly represents Christ's crown of thorns and the berries drops his of blood.[200] In northern Europe, it was believed that holly would protect one from storms, lightning, fire and the evil eye, so some people would put it above their doors; this may explain the great number of houses called Holly Cottage.[201] In some parts of England, people would put a collar of holly on their horses to keep them safe from misfortune.[202]

As well as offering protection, holly has the power to make animals return; cattle farmers would use a stick of holly, throwing it in the direction they had gone, and the animals would come home.[203]

In one strand of English lore, the holly is part of a plant couple, together with the ivy. 'Holly is a man', and the ivy is the female, goes an old saying; at some old English Shrove Tuesday a Holly Boy and an Ivy Girl were appointed.[204]

∞   **Holly in gender-related spells.** Use holly to represent male persons and ivy to represent females. It can serve as a poppet itself, or else it can decorate a poppet which you have made of wax, fabric or a mandrake or bryony root. The holly leaf or sprig is most appropriately used when it is being paired, in the spell, with a woman, who should be represented by a sprig of ivy.

∞   **Holly for space protection.** Use holly particularly for home protection against natural disaster; if you use it in this way, we recommend consecrating the holly charm with a small rite, asking the blessing of Thor, the god of thunderbolts. You might want to carve a Thurisaz rune on it, the rune of the thorn and of Thor. This and other runes are easily found online. We recommend first sweeping your house, or the place you are protecting, and sprinkling it with some herb-infused saltwater. Only then set up the spiky holly leaves around the perimeter.

∞   **Holly for personal protection.** Use holly to protect yourself against misfortune brought about by others' jealousy (the evil eye). Its sharp spikes repel malice, protecting you from it. Ask the holly plant for its assistance in protecting you, then place the leaves to form a protective perimeter. This plant is possibly the most aggressive plants used to protect against ill wishing from malicious envy. People who are wishing you failure will experience a nasty comeback, perhaps a sudden misfortune. There are other, kinder plants to use if you wish your ill-wishers to be healed of their spiritual illness, so think twice before choosing this option.

∞   **Holly for bringing pets and animals home again.** Cut a holly wand; the traditional length for a wand is from your elbow to the tip of your longest finger. Peel it immediately, before the bark sticks to the wood, ideally within two hours of cutting. Sand, and then oil it with a mixture made up of oil, a sample of your saliva or blood and one of your pet's bodily fluids. Keep the wand near the animal's sleeping place. When your pet has gone missing or run away, take the wand, stand near your home (or their stables) and sing the animal's name for about ten minutes—it is longer than it seems, so I suggest using a timer. Then throw the wand as hard and as far as you can in the direction the animal went in—or you think it went in. Then wait.

Honesty (lunary)

Also known as lunary, lunarie, lunaria; used to be known also as moonwort

Lunaria annua, Lunaria biennis. Attribution: Moon (Culpeper) This is a common wild plant with small purple flowers and seed pods which dry and resemble silvery full moons. In Southeast Asia, it is called 'money plant' and in the United States some called it 'silver dollars'. Honesty is a plant of the moon; in fact, as 'lunary', it is named for it. It is a famous magical plant in Britain and Europe, specifically as a witchcraft herb; indeed, it is a herb which should be in the kitchen of every witch. Chaucer is one of the many people who say it is one of the herbs that magicians put into their magical potions:

And herbes coud I tell eke many (much more) on
As Egremain, Valerian and Lunarie
... to bring about our craft, if that we may.[205]

The sixteenth-century writer Michael Drayton also says it
is a magical plant; he writes of a witchy woman preparing a
potion to cure madness:

Then sprinkles she the juice of Rue,
with nine drops of the midnight dew,
from Lunary distilling.[206]

Elsewhere, Drayton speaks of finding the plant growing
wild: 'Enchanting Lunarie here lies, in sorceries excelling.'[207]
But we struggle to know much about what those sorceries
might be. Honesty spells were unknown to many folklore
collectors of the nineteenth century (Friend, for example); its
use appears to have largely died out by then. One of the few
things we know is that in England it was put in potions to
'put evil to flight'.[208] Another is that it has the power to open
locks: 'moonwort will open locks wherewith dwelling-houses
are made fast, if it be put into the key-hole'.[209]

✏ **Honesty to restore spiritual equilibrium.** It 'puts
evil to flight', and this can mean evil people, your personal demons, or institutional forces of destruction. Improvise
with Drayton's recipe above to make a potion with juice of
rue, dew collected at midnight and some distilled extract of
honesty leaves. We recommend making your potion on a full
moon, the time of great magical power, which will attune to
the lunar power of the plant itself.

✏ **Honesty for unlocking doors or gaining access.** You
can use the herb in a potion to open physical doors, but you
can also use it to unblock your access to a place which you
wish to enter, for example, a university, an art school, an
invitation-only event. Use honesty in a potion or spell which
is about unlocking spaces or avenues of endeavour which are
currently closed to you.

Hyssop

Hyssopus officinalis. Attribution: Jupiter (Culpeper)

This hardy, purple-flowering shrub, native to southern Europe, is a plant which bears a slight resemblance to the lavender bush that is so common in England. In Judaism and Christianity, hyssop is a potent plant of purification and, at the same time, a symbol of God's forgiveness; this is summarised in the well-known Christian phrase from Psalm 51, used in the Mass during the sprinkling of holy water: *Asperges me Domine hyssopo et mundabor lavabis me et super nivem dealbabor* ('Thou wilt sprinkle me, O Lord, with hyssop, and I shall be cleansed. Thou wilt wash me, and I shall be washed whiter than snow.') It is thus a plant which is used to wash with, or sprinkle with, when you need purification. Using hyssop is appropriate when you need to be cleansed after you've committed a misdeed and want to cleanse yourself from shame' (after making reparation, of course). It is equally appropriate to use when you need to cleanse and reconsecrate yourself after you have been violated by another person, verbally, sexually or physically.

Hyssop is imbued with the uplifting benevolent force of Jupiter. Thus it is used against dark moods and dark forces. A famous medieval physician prescribed hyssop against melancholy; Hildegard of Bingen recommended a meal of chicken cooked in hyssop and wine as a treatment for 'sadness'.[210] In Palermo, Sicily, women go out on St Mark's Day (25 April) to gather armfuls of hyssop, which they put in their homes to keep away the evil eye.[211]

∞ **Hyssop against melancholy.** Make a chicken soup from Hildegard's recipe, above. Season your chicken soup with hyssop and cook it with a few tablespoons of white wine, and it will make a meal that is both magical and delicious. If possible, serve the soup from a purple bowl, or at a table dressed with a purple cloth: this is the colour of Jupiter, 'the great benificent', whose virtue permeates the hyssop plant. If the soup is prepared and eaten on a Thursday, so much the better.

∞ **Hyssop for space protection.** Put hyssop around you in the house or your work space. It is especially appropriate to use when you have concerns about what in earlier days would be called the evil eye, namely unpleasant energy directed towards you which arises from jealousy or envy. If possible, do this on a Thursday.

 ∾ **Hyssop for personal purification and cleansing.** Make a cup of strong hyssop tea using two tablespoons of the herb in a cup of boiling water. Run a bath, then pour the tea into the bath. Bathe in candlelight, using white candles. If you are Christian or Jewish, you may wish to recite Psalm 51 as you wash yourself.

Ivy

Genus *Hedera*. Attribution: Saturn (Culpeper)

Ivy is an evergreen plant found crawling up walls and fences and winding around trees all over England. In English folk-lore, it is a Christmas decoration, and it is generally believed it should be in the house only for that season.[212] Also in English folklore, ivy is the plant of women, and ivy represents a woman in magical spells. There is a male–female couple in plants—in this couple, the ivy is female and her male partner is the holly. In Somerset, there was around Yuletide the tradition of having a Holly Boy and an Ivy Girl.[213]

Ivy can also bring good fortune. Growing on a house, it protects it from ill.[214] It also gives the power to see who wishes one harm. One old piece of folklore says that wearing an ivy wreath—particularly on May Day—gives a person the power to 'distinguish between good women and bad', and with such a crown on one's head, the wearer will 'learn to know witches when he sees them'.[215]

In ancient Greece, many gods wore ivy in crowns, but it was especially sacred to Dionysos, whose followers were clad in ivy and whose thyrsus wands were entwined with it.[216]

 ∾ **Ivy to discern bad people.** Make an ivy crown to discern a wrong'un. This is good to do when you are uncertain of someone's character. Once you have put on the crown, you will get a distinct feeling as to whether they are a problematic person. They may suddenly do something which reveals their character, for good or ill, or you may receive some piece of information about them—a phone call or a message, for example.

∞ **Ivy in spells involving women.** Use ivy to symbolise the woman in your spell. If there is a male in the spell as well, use a sprig of holly to represent him. In spellcraft, it is a longstanding tradition to make dolls, poppets or symbolic representations of the people involved. Mandrake, bryony root, ivy and holly are the most common plants used for this.

Juniper

Also known as savin, saffern, saffron. Attribution: Sun (Culpeper)

Genus *Juniperus.*

The juniper is one of the important plants in European folk magic, used across the continent as recently as the twentieth century and all the way back to ancient Greece.[217] The juniper is a protecting, sheltering tree in several biblical stories, which may partially account for its wide and continuing recognition.[218] An old German saying is 'Oak leaf and juniper: the Devil isn't fond of them.'[219]

In medieval and early modern times juniper wood was burned for its smoke, which deters demons.[220] The Scots, right up to the nineteenth century, would burn it to ward off the evil eye.[221] British folklore says it is well known that if you have a juniper tree planted by the door to your home, a witch cannot enter.[222] In Italy, people brush juniper branches over holes and fissures in a house to prevent evil spirits entering the building.[223] Unsurprisingly, juniper should not be cut, at least in Wales: the Welsh say that whoever cuts down a juniper tree will die within the year.[224]

The juniper's spirit is petitioned in this old spell to get back a stolen item.

Juniper Finding Spell

In this spell, you must find a young juniper with a supple trunk. Bend it over to the earth in an arch, and weigh the top end down with two weights: a big stone and the skull of a murderer. Then say, 'Juniper, I bend and squeeze you till the thief [say their name here] returns what he has taken to its place.' Soon the thief will come to you and return the taken item or items. This will happen because the spell will make the person have an unstoppable urge to return the goods to you. It will occur quite quickly. When you have your goods back, you must rush back to the tree, release it from its cramped position, and give it due thanks.[225]

Juniper's helpful, protective quality is nonetheless linked to death, for in ancient Greece its green branches were burned as incense on offerings to Hades.[226] Also, it was known to be sacred to the furies, so its berries were burned at funerals to keep off demons.[227]

✑ **Juniper to bless the dead.** Burn juniper in the room or the house when someone has died. We recommend taking a few sprigs or dried berries and putting them on to a glowing charcoal in an incense burner, burning them as you would any loose resin incense. Drape your forearms with a piece of black fabric—anything will do—then circle the room with the burner, then go through the whole house, moving in a clockwise direction, so the space is infused with the scent of the juniper.

✑ **Juniper for house protection.** This is one of the most powerful plants of protection. We recommend it to clear places where bad things have happened, and also when you have a situation of the evil eye, namely unpleasant energy directed towards you which arises from jealousy or envy. Here are some ideas. Plant a juniper tree by the door of your house. Alternatively, find a local juniper tree, cut a branch from it, having asked its permission and blessing, then go home and sweep all the doorways and windowsills with it. Another way to use juniper for house protection is to dry some of its needles and berries, put them on charcoals and burn them as a magical protection incense; the smoke distributes the juniper essence through the space.

✑ **Juniper for personal protection.** Burn juniper berries as an incense, wafting the smoke around your body and breathing it gently. Alternatively, make a small bag of juniper berries and wear it around your neck. The bag should be black, as should the string you wrap it with.

∞ **Juniper to get back stolen items.** Perform the old English spell related above.

Lady's mantle

Genus *Alchemilla*. Attribution: Venus (Culpeper, Lilly)
Lady's mantle is a wild plant which grows around the British Isles and is characterised by masses of tiny yellow flowers. Scottish Highlanders say it has the power to restore a person's beauty, regardless of how much it has faded.[228]

∞ **Lady's mantle for attractiveness.** Use lady's mantle in a balm, ointment or bath which you have prepared with the intention of improving your physical attractiveness. Our recommendation is to do this on a Friday evening while the moon is waxing, or at a full moon. Set up a large mirror at a table, drape the frame with a green sash, light green candles and decorate the table with anything you own which is made of copper and any green crystals or rose quartz. Take a bath in which you've sprinkled some lady's mantle. Once you have come out, put on some gentle music, light some candles and turn out the lights. Sitting in front of the mirror, honour your body, then slowly massage the lady's mantle cream or oil into your skin, all the while asking the blessing of the plant. Adorn yourself with jewellery, cosmetics or fabric which makes you feel magnificent. The internet has instructions on how to take herbs and make them into a body oil, balm or body cream, so you can do this yourself in advance of the Friday-night ceremony.

Lemon balm

See balm

Lime tree

Also known as linden tree, line tree
Genus *Tilia*. Attribution: Jupiter/Venus; Moon (Lilly).[229]
In Germanic, Hungarian and Polish regions, the lime, or linden, is deeply sacred. A linden tree is found on the central green of almost every village in Germany; beneath it, magistrates

would sit to give their judgement on local disputes or cases, so it came to be known as the tree of judgement. Moreover, for Germans, the lime tree's holiness was also supernatural: in it and around it were where dwarfs and fairies lived and gathered.[230] The shade of the lime tree was a favourite resting place of dragons; so much so that dragons came to be known as lindenworms. Unsurprisingly, it is taboo to cut down a linden tree.[231] Many villagers will plant one in front of a new house to keep the witches from entering.[232]

In Scandinavian tradition, though, it is a tree of misfortune. In an old myth, the hero Sigurd bathed in dragon blood, which had the power of deflecting arrows. But because a lime-tree leaf lay on one spot of his shoulder at that moment, the magic blood did not protect him there, and he was stabbed. Hence the lime tree brings bad luck.[233]

The lime features in the Greek myth of Philemon and Baucis, a devoted couple who served Jove and Mercury so loyally that when they died Philemon was turned into an oak and Baucis into a linden. Because of this, the linden tree is a tree of hospitality and of conjugal love.

Scythian soothsayers turned to the linden when they were about to prophesy and wrapped its leaves about their fingers when they sought inspiration, as if it spoke to them.[234]

∞ **Linden for justice.** Use linden leaves or lime juice in potions to bring about justice. One way you can do this is to write out the problem, or collect relevant papers or material. Take them, together with some purple ribbon, out to a local linden tree on a Thursday. Once you are under the tree, invoke the justice of the linden spirit, then, with a clear, calm mind, bind the papers with the purple ribbon. Bury them under the tree, or bring them home with a twig of the linden tree; at home, keep them on your home altar or mantelpiece. Purple is the correct colour to use because it is the colour of justice and of favourable decisions from people in authority.

∞ **Linden for seeing fairies or dragons.** Visit a lime tree and sit under it. We recommend making such an outing on May Eve (Beltane) at night, or on another night when the veil between the worlds is thin, such as Midsummer's Eve or

Hallowe'en. It is good practice to bring an offering for the beings you hope to encounter, such as milk, cream or whiskey.

∾ **Linden for a happy marriage and a home full of friends.** Do a spell with lime and oak leaves. We recommend using green and gold ribbons to make a large wreath to hang on the home's front door or in the house. Green is the colour of love and gold the colour of radiant happiness. The home blessed with linden leaves will be a place where the fairies are welcome and where fairness prevails.

∾ **Linden for finding someone's vulnerable spot.** Use linden leaves in a working to find the point of vulnerability or access, when someone's shield seems impenetrable. Use the story of Sigurd as a storyline to work from.

Love-in-a-mist
Nigella damascena. Attribution: none given in either Culpeper or Lilly
This is a delicate, star-shaped garden flower, usually blue but sometimes white or pink. Folklore says that love-in-a-mist, if worn between the breasts, will draw a love to you.[235]

∾ **Love-in-a-mist for love.** Use it in a love-drawing spell, especially for women. Whatever you choose do do, ensure that its final step is to place a pouch of the flowers against your chest. As with all love charms, we recommend doing the charm on a Friday, the day of love, and using the colour green for the pouch or wrap.

Lunary
See honesty

Mandrake
Genus *Mandragora.* Attribution: Mercury (Culpeper); Saturn (Lilly)
This leafy wild plant is native to the Mediterranean and does not grow much in northern Europe or Britain. But even where it was rare, it was much sought after in folk magic, as it is the best thing to use in any spell where a poppet is called for.

Mandrakes have a similar shape to a human so they have long been the preferred root to symbolise—or actually embody—the person the magic in intended for.[236] In Britain, those who could not find, or afford, a true mandrake would make do with bryony, which came to be called English mandrake. It can be used for love as well: the plant of the mandrake (even not as a poppet) has the power to inspire love, so it is good ingredient to use in love spells.[237]

✑ **Mandrake in spells.** Carve the root into the shape of the person you are working the magic upon, and use the doll (poppet) as their stand-in. It is suggested that you mark or carve the mandrake in some way to indicate the person's identity: shape it with their features, inscribe their initials, tie it with a strand of their hair, or something similar.

Marigold
Also known as calendula.
Genus *Calendula*. Attribution: Sun (Culpeper)
Marigold, that round, sunny flower found in so many gardens, is a solar plant, with Culpeper attributing it to the sun in Leo. The garden marigold, often called the 'African Marigold', came originally from southern France and has been cultivated in England since 1570. In Western art, it was a symbol sometimes of grief (on account of a Greek myth about marigolds), but sometimes of wealth, because of its strong gold colour. In Catholicism, the marigold is associated with the Virgin May (Mary's gold).[238] In England, it is believed to give constancy in love, so it was included in wedding bouquets and love divinations.[239]

This is an old German charm to increase your sexiness and desirability. Take a purple silk handkerchief, find a growing marigold, dig it up and remove its root, then immediately wrap the root in the cloth. Keep the bundle on you when you go out into society, and people will find you attractive and be romantically drawn to you.[240]

✑ **Marigold for social success, popularity and love.** Perform the German method above. Our suggestion is to do this on a Sunday, the day when the marigold is at its most powerful. Sunrise or midday is the ideal time to pull up the root and, before doing so, you should ask the blessing of the plant spirit.

∞   **Marigold for faithfulness.** Give your beloved something containing marigolds. This could be a bouquet, or some calendula ointment (this health product, or any calendula health product, is made of the extract of marigolds). Calendula herbal tea is easily made from dried marigold flowers, which are available to buy; this tea can be shared with one's partner. One person we know puts a little bit of calendula tea in their washing machine, so both her and her partner's clothes are washed with a little bit of calendula, and this helps them stay loyal to one another.

∞   **Marigold for wealth.** Use marigold flowers in money spells. We suggest that you use the whole flower, as when they are whole they resemble gold coins. Wealth spells using marigold are best done on Sundays, the day of radiant success.

Marjoram, sweet marjoram

Origanum majorana. Attribution: Mercury (Culpeper, Lilly)
Marjoram is a cooking herb found in most kitchen cabinets, but it is also a powerful magical herb. Culpeper writes that marjoram 'is much used in all odoriferous water, powders, &c. that are for ornament or delight'. It is very much connected with sensuality, the delight of scent and lovemaking. According to Rapin, the goddess Venus cultivated marjoram, and its scent derived from the goddess's touch.[241] In ancient Greece and Rome, newly married couples were crowned with it. In England and Germany, marjoram has long been used against witchcraft, for 'no person who has sold themselves to the Devil can abide it'.[242]

∞   **Marjoram for personal protection.** Use marjoram in spells for protection of yourself, to keep toxic and dangerous people away from you. The old language is 'people who have sold their souls to the devil', meaning people who have undertaken to do harm to those they know. In modern parlance, this refers to those who wish you ill, those who would exert coercive control, and those who would take pleasure in your failure. The scent is an important part of the herb's effectiveness, so be sure that the leaves or essential oil of marjoram can work their power.

∞   **Marjoram for blessing relationships.** Make a marjoram crown for both parties. We suggest interweaving other flowers of love into the crown as well; the list at the beginning of this book will offer guidance on your options. If you use ribbon in making the crown, use ones which are green and/or pink, with red as well if you are looking to energise the crown with spicy erotic energy.

∞   **Marjoram for love.** This is a wonderful herb to use when working magic for love. We suggest a love bath with it. Use fresh leaves crushed in the bath, or, if you only have dried marjoram, sprinkle generously into the hot water, so there is a noticeably scented steam in the bathroom. The best day for love baths is Friday, the day of love. That said, you can use marjoram in other ways as well; for example, anoint your love charm with marjoram essential oil, put a bunch of marjoram next to a photo of yourself and your beloved, or make a marjoram pillow which you embroider with the initials of the two lovers.

Meadowsweet

Filipendula ulmaria. Attribution: Venus/Jupiter (Culpeper)[243] Damp meadows all across Europe have meadowsweet growing in them; it is a tall, grass-like plant with clumps of tiny, furry white flowers. The Finns use meadowsweet in a spell to reveal the identity of a thief; to do this, they make a meadowsweet herbal tea on Midsummer's Day; once you have drunk the tea, something will happen very shortly thereafter which makes it clear who that person is.[244]

∞   **Meadowsweet to detect a thief (at midsummer).** Perform the Finnish working outlined above, around the 21st of June. Our recommendations for this working: First, it is traditional to gather midsummer herbs in the morning, a little before noon: this is when they are nearest to their peak potency, which is noon, and before they start to decline in power with the sun; so after that time is nowhere near as good. When you make the herbal tea, we advise using a yellow-coloured cup or mug, as yellow has the virtue –power—of the sun, and thus revelation of hidden things. Avoid stirring the tea with a silver-coloured spoon, we suggest. Moon-coloured metals are not good to use here.

Melissa
See balm

Milfoil
See yarrow

Milk thistle
Also known as Our Lady's thistle, St Mary's thistle
Silybum marianum. Attrib: Jupiter (Culpeper), Mars (Lilly)
Milk thistle is a plant used mainly in the medicinal side of herbalism. However, it is also used magically to lift depression and bring optimism, and this is done by making the root of it into an amulet. The great herbalist Gerard wrote of the milk thistle that: 'the root, if borne about one, doth expel melancholy'.

∾   **Milk thistle against melancholy.** Make Gerard's amulet, as follows. Find a milk thistle plant, dig up the root, dry it and tie it on to a string to wear around your neck. The virtue, or power, of the root is what effects the cure from melancholy. We recommend digging up the root on a Thursday (the day of Jupiter, of success and jovial wellbeing), letting it dry for four weeks, then tying it on to a purple cord on the fourth Thursday. Thus it will have been drying for almost a month and on either side you will be working with it on the day of its presiding energy—that of Jupiter, whose colour is purple.

Mint
Genus *Mentha.* Attribution: Venus (Culpeper), Jupiter (Lilly)
This herb is loved and known by everyone, and it has been for over a thousand years. It gets its name from classical myth: Pluto fell in love with a nymph named Mintho;

Proserpine did not approve and turned the maiden into a mint plant.[245] Mint's remarkable power is that it removes the desire to fight. Alexander the Great forbade his soldiers from eating it for this reason.[246] Its additional power is the power to aid memory. In ancient Athens, its powers in this were considered so effective that students used to wear a wreath of mint while studying.[247] Mint offers protection, particularly at the time of one's death. This is recognised explicitly in both Italy and Belgium; in Flanders, its folk name is old man's herb, and it is tied to the leg of a bed as a person is dying.[248]

∞ **Mint for a truce.** Use mint in a spell to end an argument or a feud. Equally, use it in a spell to stop a disagreement from escalating into a row or a rift. We suggest serving mint tea to the person who is angry with you, if that is possible. We recommend otherwise that you make a bundle, sachet or bouquet of herbs of friendship and peace, and into this put a strand of your hair, or something of yours, as well as something of the other party. The best day for doing any of this is on a Friday, the day of friendship and love, during the time of the waxing moon.

∞ **Mint for study and exams.** Use mint in a spell to help someone who has memory problems. When making your spell, include the mint in a way that you get a good strong scent of it, for example a pillow or a steam inhalation.

Mistletoe

Viscum album. Attribution: Sun (Culpeper)

Mistletoe is known by everyone as the plant under which we share a kiss at New Year. An evergreen, it carries connotations of life surviving through the winter. In folk magic, though, it is used for protection. In many places across Britain and Europe, people hang it up around the house and barn to drive away evil spirits.[249] An English belief is that 'of one hang mistletoe about their neck, the witches can have no power over him'.[250] Worcestershire farmers offer mistletoe to the first cow that calves after the new year to keep the herd safe through the coming year.[251] In Germany and

Mistletoe

England several centuries ago, mistletoe amulets were given to children to wear for protection. But more than protection, mistletoe brings peace and hospitality to the place where it is.[252]

Mistletoe has other powers, too. Holding a stick of mistletoe, you will be able to see ghosts and talk with them. It also has the power to prevent nightmares. In addition, it can open locks, a power much loved by burglars of previous centuries.[253]

∞ **Mistletoe for protection, peace and hospitality.** Use mistletoe in a New Year's home blessing, as part of a little ceremony of your own devising. We suggest taking the sprig through the house, into every room, perhaps with a New Year's song or a carol, asking that in the coming year your home be a place of health, happiness and prosperity. There are many herbs which are used for house and space protection, but mistletoe is especially appropriate if yours is a family home.

∞ **Mistletoe for a child blessing.** Make a mistletoe amulet for a child you are fond of, as its power is that of protection; it was traditionally given to children in this form to keep them safe.

∞ **Mistletoe to communicate with ghosts.** Carve a wand of mistletoe and hold it in order to perceive the spirits of the dead.

∞ **Mistletoe for opening locks.** Use the dried herb for this. Mix it in a potion to unlock literal doors, but also to gain access to institutions and meetings which are gate-kept. For example, you can use mistletoe if you are desperate to get an invitation to a meeting at which you can make a big difference, or pitch a career-changing proposal. As so much contact is made these days via the internet, consider waving a branch of mistletoe over the message you hope will get you 'through the door'. On your altar or on special table, place mistletoe around an item symbolising the place to which you are determined to gain entry.

Motherwort

Leonurus cardiaca. Attribution: Venus (Culpeper)

This hardy, invasive plant which grows on the roadsides and in overgrown gardens is not much used in herb magic spells, but when it does appear it shows a wonderful power: it causes the person bearing it to be able to run supernaturally fast. We learn this power from an old spell in which one fashioned garters of hare skin, then infused them with motherwort. When the wearer began to move, he or she 'could outrun horses'.

∞ **Motherwort for speed in athletics and running.** Perform a modernised variant of the motherwort spell above to help an athlete increase their speed. Soak clothes, socks or even running shoes in water infused with motherwort. Dry them, then give them to the athlete. When they run, they will achieve better speed times than they have ever done before. Alternatively, you can make a powder of dried motherwort and sprinkle a few pinches into the shoes of the athlete, ideally doing so on a Wednesday, which is the day of the god of swiftness, Mercury.

Mugwort

Also known as artemisia.

Artemesia vulgaris. Attribution: Venus (Culpeper, Lilly)

In European and British folk magic, this is one of the most important of all magical plants. It is a bushy wild plant which grows tall, with leaves that have a distinctively silver underside. It grows in verges, unkempt areas and open grasslands. In folk magic, mugwort appears over and over again, attributed with great powers. In Germany, it is called 'Mother of All Herbs'. As far back as late-Roman times, it was known to keep one safe: Apuleius said it drove away demons.[254] And the belief has persisted into modern times. Examples abound from all across Europe.[255] To give one example in Somerset, an old man in 1906 told a folklore collector that, with mugwort, 'If yew do pick'n right, there idn't nothing you can't wish vor.'[256]

The plant's official name derives from the huntress goddess Artemis, and the plant is sacred to her.[257] For the Greeks and Romans, the association of mugwort to Artemis/Diana did not extend so far as chastity. The Greeks and Romans used it as an aphrodisiac charm which they would place under the bed before an erotic encounter they wanted to go well.[258]

Mugwort's love powers are widely recognised. To attract a lover, people wear a little sprig of it; women are sometimes told to keep some between their breasts. Couples use it to protect their relationship from the evil spirits which attack committed relationships.[259]

Perhaps because she was a tireless huntress, Artemis's herb has the power to energise people while walking or running, whether they be in the woods chasing wild animals or doing a ten-mile trek. In ancient Rome, soldiers wore mugwort in their sandals during long marches to give them continued strength. The belief carried on into English folklore; as late as the twentieth century, it was widely known that, in a shoe sole, mugwort prevents weariness.[260]

Mugwort is one of the St John's herbs gathered at midsummer for magic. In fact, in the Netherlands and Germany, one of its names is St John's Plant.[261] If picked at their right time, the plants sacred to St John afford protection against bad luck and evil. In one variant of this belief, it is said that a crown made from its sprays was worn on St John's Eve (Midsummer's Eve) to give the wearer protection against being possessed by evil.[262] Mugwort's association with St John is also evident in its medieval alternative name, *Cingulum Sancti Johannis* ('the belt of St John'), and one old story claims that when John the Baptist was in the wilderness he wore a belt of mugwort around his waist.[263]

A nineteenth-century French writer gives this recipe for such a belt, in which you pick stems of mugwort, then steep them in a jar of a young girl's urine. After three days, remove them, let them dry, then enclose them into a belt of some sort. This belt will afford wondrous protection.[264] Mugwort is a powerful protection at all times, however, not just at midsummer. An old German charm for safety against evil forces can be done at any time: make three bouquets of the herb and put them around your room.[265]

✎ **Mugwort for protection.** Best to do such a working at the summer solstice, but you can do it any time. Make a protection belt or a protection crown, in line with the old customs. We suggest picking midsummer herbs (those traditionally gathered at that time) before noon on the day of the summer solstice or on the Day of St John (24 June). If you are pagan, you may wish to keep to the astronomical solstice, whereas if you are Christian, St John's Day might feel more right to you. The reason for picking the herbs in the morning is to be sure of catching them while the year's energy is still peaking, and before the energy of decline sets in, as it does from the minute the solstice is past—or from the passing of the middle of the day.

∞ **Mugwort for travellers' energy.** Use mugwort in a shoe spell for untiring foot travel. Make a flat envelope of mugwort, then put it in your shoe before you set out on an important walk. Another way to get the same effect is to grind a few teaspoons of dried mugwort into a fine powder and place some on the insides of each shoe. As you prepare the mugwort, whichever way you choose, we recommend speaking to the plant's spirit to ask it to bless the traveller. The best day to do this is a Wednesday, the day of the god of travel (Mercury).

∞ **Mugwort for good sex.** Mugwort is particularly good for women, due to the connection with Artemis. Place some mugwort under your bed, if you wish to use it in the most traditional way. Alternatively, we suggest adding it to a bouquet of sex-enchancing flowers and leaves to place in the bedroom or wherever your seduction will take place. A small pillow of dried mugwort and other herbs is a good way to get the same result; we suggest using green fabric, the colour of Venus, or red, the colour of drive and passion.

∞ **Mugwort for women athletes.** Employ the herb in a charm and it will give women extra speed and endurance. One way to do this is to make a powder of dried mugwort and ceremonially sprinkle some of the powder into their running shoes, doing so on a night of the full moon, as the magic is powerful then, and it is also under the full moon that hunters such as the goddess Artemis would run through the woods after their prey.

Myrtle, flowering

Genus *Myrtus*. Attribution: Mercury (Culpeper)
Myrtle, a delicate purple or pink wildflower, is often over-looked in herbal magic, but it has wonderful powers. It is a plant of Venus, whose temples were planted around with myrtle; her attendants, the Graces, wore crowns of it. During Venus's May festivals, married couples would wear myrtle wreaths. Its magical power is that it encourages sensual grat-ification. 'When the festival of the Bona Dea came around, it was allowable for the Romans to use every plant, flower, and leaf in the decorations, save only the myrtle, which was barred on the ground that it encouraged sensuality.'[266]

Somerset people believe a flowering myrtle is the greatest acquisition a house can have, but one has to treat it properly. The owner must show his pride in it all the time. The attitude of pride must commence from the outset of your relationship with the plant. You should spread out the skirt of your dress when you put the slip in a pot to start it growing, and look proud! You must keep it your window where others can see it, and you must water it every day, to show your pride in it. Any other things to show your pride in it will help. If you do all these things, the myrtle will make your home and family outstandingly fortunate, blessed, wealthy and happy.[267]

∾   **Myrtle for good sex.** Use myrtle flowers and leaves in your spells or bath to encourage sensuality. Put a bunch of myrtle flowers in a small vase by your bed, or give a bouquet with myrtle to your sweetheart.

∾   **Myrtle for a happy and prosperous home.** Plant a myrtle at home, following the Somerset instructions for showing pride in it above, ideally from a slip you've acquired, so that you have a relationship with the plant from its beginnings. Remember to show the world you are proud of it, to praise it and show it off. The spirit of the plant will give great blessings to the household.

Narcissus

See daffodil

Oak

Genus *Quercus*. Attribution: Jupiter (Culpeper, Lilly).

The oak belongs to Jupiter; it is by agreement the tree of the god by his many names and regional aspects, be it Jove or Thor.[268] It is widely used, since ancient times to the present, for good fortune and protection from harm and evil.[269] It is the archetypal royal tree, king of the woods: as such, oaks were worshipped in pagan times and they were considered givers of protection through the Middle Ages and beyond. When Christianity came, the fairies went to live in the oaks, where they live to this day. The doors to the oak-tree dwelling are the holes on the trunk caused by fallen branches. These are known as 'fairy doors'. To call to the oak-dwelling fairies, rub your hand on the hole; this is the equivalent of knocking on their door. Do this always with courtesy, whether you are doing it simply to honour them or to contact them to ask their blessing and help. If you have something needing healing or blessing, rub it against the fairy door.[270] Some say that when petitioning an oak for help you should make an offering to it of a lock of hair.[271] It is said that fairies dance around Herne's Oak in Windsor Great Park.

> The fairies, from their nightly haunt,
> In copse or dell, or round the trunk revered
> of Herne's moon-silvered oak, shall chase away
> Each fog, each blight, and dedicate to peace
> Thy classic shade.[272]

In England's West Country, the oak is chosen to be the Yule log at Christmas (or sometimes apple): oak is chosen for 'strength in the maister and safety from thunder', while apple is chosen to bring good luck—the Yule log must be burned on all of the twelve days of Christmas.[273]

∽ **Oak for protection and good fortune.** Oak is particularly appropriate to use for protection when you are protecting your position of authority, or your power over your domain. The oak is the king of the forest, in old lore, and his kindred gods are Jupiter and Thor, older father gods who are bearers of lightning bolts. Use oak bark or oak leaves in spells, for example, for an older man whose children are trying to get him to sign over his house to them. Or for a woman CEO who is the victim of a plot to oust her, or a founder of a family business losing money because of illness or lack of support from family members.

✀   **Oak for inner or physical strength.** Use oak bark or oak leaves. Oak is a great tree to call upon, with bark or leaf, when you are doing a spell to give a leader strength, solidity and resolve. One would use this to do a spell to support one's senator, MP, or elected representative when they are standing up for a cause you care about. You can use it for yourself, too, particularly when speaking out and advocating for justice.

✀   **Oak for strength through the whole year.** Burn an oak Yule log at Christmas or, if you prefer, at the winter solstice. It is worth remembering that you can do this not only in a fireplace but also outside, an option if you don't have a fireplace in your home. If it's not feasible for you to burn a log, you can burn a smaller branch or even a twig. We recommend preparing the oak before burning it: speak to the oak spirit, ask its blessing, douse it with an alcoholic drink and tie it with red ribbon, focussing on the quality of strength as you do so. Red is the colour of fortitude (Mars), which is why we suggest that colour.

✀   **Oak to gain favours from fairies.** Perform fairy-door petitions on oak trees, as outlined above. We recommend locating your local oak trees, then scouting them out to establish which has a fairy door. Then, when you are in need of help, you'll know exactly where to go. When you do need the fairies' help, we suggest not only acting courteously and leaving a lock of hair, as the folklore advises, but also leaving an offering. It is well known the fairies like milk, cream and alcoholic drinks. As for timing, we advise making the petitions on the fairy doors either at sunrise, sunset, midday or midnight.

✀   **To meet the oak-tree spirits or fairies.** Dance around an old oak tree, in sympathy with the fairies' custom of dancing around Herne's oak. If you wish to do this with friends, you can combine it with a picnic and invite people to bring musical instruments. If you do this on your own, we recommend preparing ahead which songs you wish to sing and dancing solo to the sound of your own voice.

Olive tree

Olea europaea. Attribution: Jupiter (Culpeper);[274] Sun, Jupiter (Lilly)

The olive is sacred to Athena, who is the goddess of cities. In Italy, it is used for house protection: a branch of olive is placed above the door to keep out 'devils and wizards'.[275]

∽ **Olive for house protection, especially in cities.** Use olive leaves in a house-protection spell for city dwellings. To do this, take some sprigs and tie them with yellow ribbon, the colour of the sun, which is their dominant essence. Hang the bunch above your front door.

∽ **Olive for personal protection in the city.** As Athena is the goddess of cities, and as this is her plant, she protects all who carry it in urban areas. Make a little bag or wrap of olive leaves, using yellow thread; in the wrap include a slip of paper on to which you've drawn two owl eyes, the eyes of the bird sacred to the goddess.

Pansy

Also known as heart's ease, love-in-idleness

Viola tricolor. Attribution: Saturn (Culpeper)[276]

Pansy's cheerful flower has an association with love which goes way back: Romans said the pansy was white until hit by Cupid's arrow, whereupon it turned purple. Pansy can cause someone to fall in love suddenly. In Shakespeare's *A Midsummer Night's Dream,* it is pansy juice that's rubbed on Titania's eyes to make her fall for the first-comer. Magically, it is a quick-acting plant and it arouses frisky desire rapidly.[277] This is indicated in its folk names: cuddle-me, kiss-me-quick, call-me-to-you, Johnny-jump-up-and-kiss-me. Another of its wonderful qualities is that it cures heartache. Again, the clue lies in its folk-names, which include heart's ease.'

∞ **Pansy for heart-healing.** Use pansy in heartache spells, for its power is indicated in its folk names: heart's ease. We recommend using pansy to help heartbreak in the following way. Pick the flowers on Monday, the day of feelings and tears, the 'moon day'. Alternatively, pick them when the moon is waning, as this is the time of the month when things more easily diminish and fade—in this case, one's deep pain and unhappy love. Once you have the pansies, put them in a ring around a photograph of yourself, which you have placed upon a yellow fabric (yellow being the colour of wellbeing): thus you will have created a mandala of your own healing. In addition, we recommend taking a candle-lit bath into which you have sprinkled pansy petals, with the bathroom lit by only yellow candles.

∞ **Pansy for love and sex, quickly achieved.** Use in love spells when a speedy result is wanted and the goal is infatuated lovemaking. On a Friday, the day of love, collect pansies and crush them to release their juice; mix the resulting 'mash' with a little unscented moisturising cream. If possible, find an excuse to rub this on to the eyelids of the person with whom you wish to have a passionate love affair. If this is not possible, use your initiative to find a way to get them to put the cream on to their skin—perhaps offer it as a hand cream. Be sure you are the first person they will see after they have done this, for this is who they will desire. Another approach is to make a salad, then sprinkle on it some pansy petals; they are edible. Serve the leafy dish to the object of your affections while you are present, so that they are gazing at you when the pansy takes effect. It is generally considered unethical to perform love magic on another person without their agreement, so we recommend always asking first. If you want to help yourself fall head over heels with a person, you can make the cream, or the salad, for yourself.

Parsley (wild celery)
Apium graveolens. Attribution: Mercury (Culpeper)
Lore also applies to closely related plants that are often called parsley, that is, smallage (wild celery).

Parsley is widely recognised as having powers of protection, as do two very similar plants, smallage and wild celery. Bits of parsley are stuffed in the cracks of barns to keep the animals inside safe from misfortune. In the south of France, a way of undoing a curse is to give the victim a herbal tea made from parsley and holy water. Elsewhere, it is traditional to carry a bit of parsley to keep evil away. In some places, farmers give parsley to their animals to eat for the same reason. It has also long been believed that parsley is an aphrodisiac so, by extension, it has powers to keep your partner interested in you and faithful to you. In one part of Germany, people would wear a bit of parsley in their clothing to keep their partners from cheating on them.[278]

∾ **Parsley for personal protection.** Use parsley for protection in any way you can think of: eat it, drink it in tea, carry small amounts in your bag or clothing. It is especially recommended to use parsley for personal protection when you are concerned about your relationship.

∾ **Parsley for home protection.** Put pinches of the dried herb at the doors and windows, or bunches of fresh parsley over your doorways and windows. There are many herbs used for house protection in Britain and Europe, so you have an option of choosing a plant which has other powers as well.

∾ **Parsley for faithfulness.** To keep your partner sexually loyal to you, sprinkle pinches of dried parsley in your spell-working mixtures when you are doing magic for the relationship. Another method is to put a pinch of parsley into a wrap or bag, with a small piece of paper with your entwined initials; put the wrap into their luggage, coat pocket or bag.

Peony
Paeonia offinalis. Attribution: Sun (Culpeper, Lilly), Jupiter (Lilly)
Peony, a beautiful wildflower, is sacred to physicians; its name is derived from the name of Paeon, the sacred physician of Greek myth. In one version, Paeon was in fact Apollo under a different name, and healed the gods wounded in the

Trojan War. In another, Paeon was a mortal physician who cured Pluto, who, in thanks, gave him eternal life. Early doctors of medicine were known as *paeony*. Peony root appears several times in folk magic, with great powers attributed to it. In late Roman times, it was used to cure mental illness: the remedy is to place a peony flower on the sufferer while they sleep; they will be fully cured by the time they awaken. Similarly, peony was carried around to prevent any attacks of mental illness, and it was a method sworn to work.[279]

Peony was used to drive out demons in Greek regions in the medieval period. The technique is to dry a peony root then burn it on charcoal, much as one would loose incense. The smoke releases the root's powers and it will banish all evil. The same text gives an alternative, which is to drink peony-root tea, which will banish misfortune and evil spirits from the person drinking it. Just carrying peony root in your pocket will keep you safe from bothersome spirits or ghosts.[280]

The protective power of peony root is attested in early modern England, where people wore dried peony root around their necks to keep them safe from evil spirits ('the incubus, which we call "the mare"').[281] As late as 1900, Sussex peasants did something similar, making strings of beads carved from peony roots to put around their children's necks to keep them safe from evil spirits.[282]

∞   **Peony for banishing evil, and for personal protection.** Pick a peony, asking the blessing of the plant, then wear it as you go about the day. If you have some time to spare, try this, more elaborate method: on a Sunday or a Wednesday, take a bath, dress in yellow clothes, put on any gold jewellery you own, light yellow candles, then make peony-root tea. Burn some peony root on charcoals in an incense burner, so the scent from the smoke fills the room. Drink it while saying prayers or affirmations of your faith.

∞   **Peony for a baby blessing.** Use peony root in a protection necklace for a baby or child. Thread the peony root beads on to a yellow or gold thread. It is not safe for babies to wear such a necklace, so we recommend giving it to the parents to hang in the baby's room, either in a corner or over the door.

∞   **Peony for blessings on doctors.** Use peony in spells to help a person who is in the medical profession.

Periwinkle

Genus *Vinca*. Attribution: Venus (Culpeper)

An English folk name for the periwinkle is sorcerer's violet, its French name is *violette des sorciers*, and the Italians call it *centocchio*, 'a hundred eyes'.[283] All these societies know periwinkle to have supernatural powers which make it the especial herb of sorcerers, witches and cunning folk.[284] Magicians use periwinkle to protect people from bad magic and the evil eye. So, it is a plant of magical power and healing witchcraft.[285] It is a true classic. An old Belgian saying summarises this particularly well: *Perveche contre tout mal prend sa revanche* ('Periwinkle takes revenge against anything bad').[286]

For protection, one old custom suggests wearing it as an amulet around your neck.[287] To undo psychic attack or a curse, there is an old remedy—namely, to put some periwinkle in hot water and drink it as a herbal tea.[288] It was used for people suffering from nightmares, or other psychic disturbances to their mental equilibrium.[289] Farmers put bunches of it above the doors and windows of their barns to keep their animals safe from evil forces of disease and bad luck.[290]

Periwinkle also has a secondary power, and that is the power to make people fall in love. *The Book of Secrets* (attributed to Albertus Magnus) suggests making a powder of dried houseleek and dried periwinkle; sprinkle this blend into the food the two will eat together, and romantic feelings will surely be kindled between them.[291] Nicholas Culpeper in his famous herbal says that periwinkle on its own will have the same effect. 'Periwinkle leaves eaten by man and wife together cause love—which is a rare quality indeed, if it be true.'

∞   **Periwinkle for magical power.** Use periwinkle in any spell which you create to empower yourself as a witch or magician. We recommend doing it on the full moon, at midnight, placing the periwinkle on a surface on which you have drawn a large pentagram, the symbol of magic.

✐ **Periwinkle for protection.** Use periwinkle also in spells protecting you from ill luck and the evil eye, as the sorcerers in the plant's name do. What folklore calls the evil eye is the bad luck which comes from another person's jealousy being directed towards you. Herbs which are effective against the evil eye are the ones to use when you know that you have something which arouses other people's malicious envy. With periwinkle, when it is being prepared for protecting a person from this, the old methods are to make it into an amulet to wear and to put bunches of it around your house or workplace. It is important to put the periwinkle near the thing in your life which arouses the ill will.

✐ **Periwinkle against nightmares and psychic imbalance.** Use periwinkle in spells to counteract disturbances to spiritual equilibrium. To do this, it is best to put it around the place of sleep, for it is during sleep that the mind does most of its healing and the body does most of its restoration. Magically, it is the time when the moon guides our psyches, and she is the ruler of dreams and emotions. We suggest making a pillow of periwinkle to place under the pillow during the night. The fabric should be blue or silver in colour.

✐ **Periwinkle for rekindling love.** Use periwinkle with houseleek in a powder to help two people fall in love or to revive the romantic spark between them. To do this, get the periwinkle, dry it, then grind it into a powder. Do the same with houseleek. Mix the two, then put a tiny pinch of it into the shared food of the couple you are helping. Alternatively, use periwinkle leaves on their own. If it is possible, light green candles to burn on the dinner table during the meal and serve the meal on green plates, or on a table dressed with a green tablecloth. It is suggested, too, to put a small bouquet of roses on the table.

Pimpernel

Genus *Anagallis*. Attribution: Sun (Culpeper), Jupiter (Lilly)
Pimpernel is a wildflower, low growing, with small pale red or blue flowers. It is a minor character in folk magic, known for one thing: its ability is to prevent evil magic from

reaching its intended victim.[292] Any pimpernel will do, but best of all is pimpernel gathered with a charm, which is addressed to the spirit of the plant:

> Herb pimpernel I have thee found
> Growing upon Christ Jesus' ground
> The same gift the Lord Jesus gave unto thee
> When He shed His blood upon the tree:
> Arise up pimpernel and go with me, And God bless me
> And all that shall wear thee. Amen.[293]

This charm should be recited 'fifteen days together, twice a day', first in the morning before breakfast, and again in the evening after having eaten one's evening meal. The charm implies that the pimpernel, once plucked, should then be worn by the person who is seeking its blessing. Another remarkable power of pimpernel is that it will give you second sight if you hold it in your hand.[294]

∞　**Pimpernel for protection.** Carry out an improvised version of the rite above, using your creativity. When you have plucked the pimpernel, we suggest that you prepare it into an amulet on a Sunday, the day of the sun, the force of radiant wellbeing. You might put the flower into a little yellow charm bag or enclose it in a gold locket. Into the bag or locket you can also put a small slip of paper with your initials, or those of the person the amulet is for.

Pine

Also known as pitch tree.

Genus *Pinus*. Attribution: Mars/Sun (Culpeper). Jupiter/ Saturn (Lilly)[295]

In ancient Greece and Rome, the pine has the power of eternal life, so sometimes it was seen at funerals: thus, for example, a pine cone was placed upon the mausoleum of Hadrian. Similarly, in ancient Egypt, a pine cone was often placed on monuments to Osiris. Perhaps the connection to life is the source of the old folk belief that pine cones collected at midsummer make a person bulletproof.[296] There is also a connection to the sea:

pine cones float, so for this reason the ancient Greeks held the pine to be sacred to Poseidon.[297]

Pine cones are phallic in shape and so are associated with male potency and sexual drive. The Greeks and Romans linked pine with love, lust and fertility: pine cones tip the thyrsus wands of the maenads. The Greeks also believed pine was the mistress of Pan (as well as of Boreas, the wind).[298] In the Orphic mysteries, the pine cone symbolised the heart of Zagreus. And as with sex, so with fertility. The fertility resulting from the sex is evidenced in the lore of Germanic regions. As late as 1950, in Tyrol a pine tree was planted when a couple got married. In parts of Germany, a fir was planted by the door of a house where a wedding was taking place.

In Germanic areas, pines have been believed since ancient times to house spirits, and much lore abounds about them; the most well-known expression of this survives in the custom of the Christmas tree. In Germany and Sweden, it was believed that this pine is a female spirit, maternal in nature. She bears girl children, little baby spirits. And most uncanny of all, 'every hole and knot in the trunk is the point from which a wood spirit escaped into the outer world, sometimes growing and becoming as other women'.[299]

∞ **Pine for sea safety.** Use pine cones or parts of pine cones in a charm for people who are going sailing, swimming or otherwise encountering the sea. We recommend making a bundle to hang in the boat or ship. It can include other floating items, such as corks; if you use string, rope, thread or fabric, it should be blue or silver, the colours of the moon, for it is the moon who controls the sea's tides and it is the moon goddess who looks favourably upon sailors. If you are using any metal, use silver, for it is the moon's metal.

∞ **Pine for bulletproofing.** The easiest method is infusing a literal bulletproof vest. On a Tuesday (the day sacred to soldiers and those who bear arms), take some pine-resin incense (colophony) and put it on to charcoals to make a thick smoke, then waft your bulletproof vest through the smoke so it absorbs the essence of the pine. Another technique is to make a pine necklace. On a Tuesday, take a pine cone, break off the seed scales, then thread them on to a red thread or a wire; this can be as basic or as artistic as you like. You may not finish your necklace that day, which is fine, but do be sure to start it on a Tuesday. Also on a Tuesday, present it to the person you are making it for and place it around their neck in person, if that is at all possible—this last point is to help the energy of your effort go into the necklace to give it further power.

∽ **Communicating with pine-tree spirits.** Perform tree-spirit rites at pine trees.

∽ **Pine for blessing the dead.** Use pine in rituals and spells concerning eternal, or returning, life. For this, we suggest burning pine-resin incense in front of a photograph of the person, or in front of their cremated remains. Use black and white candles, for these are the colours of death and eternal life. Alternatively, if you are choosing decorations for a funeral, you can choose to adorn the coffin with pine branches and burn pine-resin incense. If you are fortunate enough to have a home with an open fire, gather your family and friends one evening and burn pine logs in the fireplace as you share memories of the departed loved one.

∽ **Pine for sex.** Use pine cones in sex spells, particularly those involving men. If you are collecting the pine cones, we recommend doing so on a Friday or a Tuesday. Sex spells are best done on Fridays, the day of love, or on Tuesdays, the day of assertion and passion. Place the pine cone, upright, in front of a picture of the person whose sex life you are helping. If you don't have a picture, you can use something that has a connection to that person: a piece of their clothing, a finger-nail, a strand of hair. Less good, but better than nothing, is something they have touched. Burn red candles.

Pomegranate
Punica granatum. Attribution: Mercury/Sun (Culpeper);[300] Jupiter (Lilly)
The pomegranate is the fruit Persephone ate in the underworld and, because she ate it, she had to return there for half the

year—hence the seasons. Taking our cue from this goddess, then, pomegranate is a fruit one should eat if trying to go to an underworld-type place or state of mind. Seventeenth-century London lore advises carrying a bit of pomegranate if you are in danger of witchcraft; if you do so, you will be perfectly free of it.[301]

∞ **Pomegranates for luck underground.** It should be used in cases, for example, for a person going cave-exploring, or else for someone who wants good luck in renovating a basement. It is a perfect protection gift for a person who is (or wants to be) a miner, a subway conductor or an Underground tube driver.

∞ **Pomegranates against evil magic.** If you are in danger of the negativity arising from ill wishing, carry a bit of pomegranate with you in your pocket. It will be especially effective if you are a person who has a connection with the underworld, for the goddess of the underworld, Persephone, will recognise you as one of her own.

Poplar

Genus *Populus*. Attribution of both white and black poplar: Saturn (Culpeper)

The poplar is a large, magnificent tree that stands grandly in the landscape and offers lots of shade. The tree has two main varieties, the white poplar and the black poplar. In both ancient and Christian myth and lore, the poplar is a tree of betrayal.[302] In spite of this negative lore, however, it does appear in at least one spell for protection against psychic attack, a working which he would perform for a client found in the records of an English cunning man. It requires getting the buds from a poplar tree beforehand:

English Cunning Man's Anti-Witchcraft Spell

With the client close by, so that no one may see her while you do this working. Then with no one watching or knowing what you do, do the following. Boil up the party's water [the client's urine]. Put in two drams of poplar bud oil [pompilion]. Then take a red-hot iron and plunge it into the pan of urine and oil, saying three times, 'In the name of the Father, the

Son and the Holy Ghost, avoid all witches and wicked person from this party, from this time forth, forevermore.'[303]

∞ **Poplar for matters concerning betrayal.** Use in spells and workings when you are being betrayed. You can also use it in situations where you are considering betraying a person, or when you find you have plans to betray a company or an institution. Betrayal can include leaking a secret to a person's enemy, cheating on a romantic partner, revealing private information to the press, or whistleblowing on unethical practice for the greater safety of workers. It can be breaking a non-disclosure agreement which binds you to keep damaging information secret. Sometimes people are sworn to secrecy to keep terrible secrets, which should be revealed to the authorities in order to protect the vulnerable. For this reason, sometimes betrayal is not a morally bad act but a good one. For magical workings dealing with betrayal, we suggest cutting a stick of poplar from a tree in your area, on a Saturday. Wrap it in a black cloth and, that night, bury it behind where you live after performing the spell.

∞ **Poplar for protection.** Perform the cunning man's spell above.

Poppy

Papaver somniferum. Attribution: Moon (Culpeper), Saturn (Lilly)
Poppy, most distinctive in the English landscape, with its red flowers in the cornfields, is of course the plant which gives us opium. It is, in folk magic—as in medicine—a plant of dreams and visions. It is also a plant of pain relief and sleep. Where sightings of the supernatural or images of strange, otherworldly beings are sought, then poppy is used. One of its related powers is the power to inspire love.[304] The love it inspires will of course be in line with the poppy's character. It will be a dreamy, languorous affair.

∞ **Poppy for love.** Use in love spells, ideally on a Friday or at the full moon. We recommend that you create a symbol which represents your state of mind when you are fulfilled in love, then, in a small, personal ceremony, trace out this shape using poppy seeds, doing so on a green surface, perhaps green cake icing on a poppy-seed and rose cake (see rose). Eat the cake in the light of green candles.

∞ **Poppy in spells for dreams and visions.** Use poppy seeds in spells to develop clairvoyance and to propitiate the forces of pain relief. Poppy seeds do not contain the narcotic effects opium does, so their use is magical rather than medical. For a spell to help you have psychic dreams and visions, we recommend baking poppy-seed muffins or cakes on a Monday, the day of the moon and dreaming. Eat a cake before going into a long sleep, ensuring you don't need to wake up early the next morning. Next to your bed we suggest putting a bunch of poppy flowers, and that you ask the poppy to give you vivid, true dreams.

Primrose

Primula vulgaris. Attribution: Venus (Culpeper)

The distinctive pale yellow flowers of this low-growing plant are a common sight around Europe, and the primrose is a much-loved part of the countryside foliage. In Germany, it is known that the primrose has the power to open up doorways to fairy caves which have riches in them. In a related belief, German lore says the goddess Bertha used primrose to lure children away from their homes and into her enchanted halls. In Somerset, primroses are carried when seeking treasure or trying to penetrate the haunts of fairies, but you must use the right number, at the right time.[305] If a child ate primroses, they would see fairies, many people believed.[306]

In Somerset, primroses are used for protection on Midsummer's Eve.[307] But in many areas, it was on May Eve (Beltane) that people put them up to protect their homes. Again in Somerset, it is customary to hang a ball of primrose over the threshold on that night.[308] On that same night in Ireland, balls of the flowers are tied to cows' tails to protect them from supernatural spirits which might be flying around. In Yorkshire, the May Eve custom is to hang up a wreath of primroses, buttercups and green leaves, for luck and protection through the coming season: the wreath is not taken down but left to wither naturally.[309]

∽　**Primrose in magic concerning mining.** Use primrose in a spell where you are trying to gain access to treasure caverns in hills. In modern times, this means you are most likely to be doing a spell for a friend who is working in mining or mineral exploration. We suggest taking a map of the area in question, surrounding it with candles and appropriate sigils and words you've written, then sprinkling primroses on to the map. Within a short while, the treasure or precious objects will be discovered or revealed. As with all plants used in spells, the primroses should first be addressed and thanked for the assistance they will give.

∽　**Primrose for protection.** Hang up primroses around you, especially on May Day or at midsummer. You can make the Yorkshire wreath described above, or little balls of primroses to hang on doorknobs or anything that swings or swishes.

∽　**Primrose for entering fairy realms or seeing fairies.** Carry primroses when you undertake an adventure to see fairies. If you want to see fairies, we recommend going out to the wildest and least busy nature area near you, looking particularly for groves of sheltering trees which have hidden overgrown patches; tradition says these are the kinds of places the fairies tend to live. (There, and in thyme bushes when they grow together in a patch, or bank.) Primroses, however, seem to be associated especially with the fairies of caves and mountains, so if your area is hilly or mountainous, these are the plants to carry when you go out looking. We always recommend doing such an expedition on a full moon or on an old day of supernatural power: May Eve, Midsummer's Morning, Lammas Eve, or Hallowe'en. If going on a physical expedition to see fairies is not to your taste, you can undertake to meet them in dreams or reverie; if you choose this method, put a bunch of primroses by your pillow and breathe in their scent as you drift off.

Purslane

Portulaca oleracea. Attribution: Moon (Culpeper)

Purslane is a low-growing herb with succulent, spoon-shaped leaves; it used to be eaten in salads. As a magical plant, it offers protection against attack by evil spirits. Strewn around one's bed, it protects against 'blastings by lightning or planets, and burning of gunpowder'.[310] Another set of old traditions says that purslane has the power to inspire love.[311]

∞   **Purslane for protection.** Use purslane when you are concerned about an explosive attack, be it from nature, from unseen forces or from human violence. The traditional method, outlined above, is to sprinkle it around your bed. If you do this, we recommend making sure you sprinkle it all the way around the bed, making sure not to omit the head of the bed; you want to be sleeping within a circle of purslane.

∞   **Purslane for love.** Use purslane in your workings of love magic. For this, we recommend finding fresh purslane and using it in a salad which you eat ceremoniously on a Friday night, Friday being the best day of the week on which to do love magic. Into the salad you might wish to add small bits of apple and other nuts, fruits and leaves with love-drawing powers.

Ragwort

Also known as ragweed. Attribution: Venus (Culpeper)

Jacobaea vulgaris and *Senecio jacobaea*

Ragwort is a well-known weed of pastures and waste ground, tall and bearing yellow flowers. In Ireland, it is believed that witches and fairies ride on it as if it were a horse, flying through the air at night; thus they call it 'fairies' horse'.[312] In Cornwall, it is believed that witches near Castle Peak gather ragweed by night for their brooms. Skinner relates it poetically:

> If ever you are in that wild part of Cornwall where Castle Peak lords it over the moors, a new experience awaits you, if you dare to stay out late. Choose some night when a harsh wind is blowing, and clouds are skurrying

across the moon: then you shall see gray, misty figures stealing over the heath. They are witches, gathering rag-weed. When they have picked a bunch of strong stems the hags bestride them and off they go, flying faster than the clouds and mixing with them as the ride goes forward to Castle Peak. If you follow, you shall see them gathered at its top, dancing, mingling in obscene worship, or brewing poisons and compounding spells.[313]

It is not used in traditional folk spells, but it does form part of the plant lore of the countryside and forms a link with the witches, their freedom of flight and their uncontrolled nature.

∞   **Rag-weed for magic.** Use it in spells in which you wish to evoke the power of witches flying across the night sky.

Rose

Genus *Rosaceae*. Attribution: Venus (this attribution is universal) Roses are famously ruled by Venus, and their history and lore is voluminous, ranging from ancient Greece and Rome to societies around the world.[314] In England, roses bloom at the height of summer; the rose is a midsummer flower.[315] Being Venusian, they are the flower of love, but carnal love rather than spiritual love. Roses were repudiated by early Christians due to their pagan associations, and they were avoided by Christians until the Middle Ages, as they brought on voluptuousness and cupidity.[316]

Roses are not often used in folk spells of Europe or the British Isles. There is, however, a Somerset love spell involving roses. On Midsummer's Day, as the clock strikes noon, pluck a white rose. Wrap it in white paper and let it dry. On Christmas Day, six months later, put it in your bosom. 'Your future husband will snatch it away.'[317] In some parts of Belgium, it is a custom to make a necklace of rose hips for children, to keep them safe from demonic forces.[318]

Roses are a symbol of silence and a command to silence: things that are spoken of underneath these flowers are kept secret and are *sub rosa*, 'under the rose'.

∽ **Rose for love.** Use rose in workings for erotic and romantic love. The oldest way is to give your beloved a dozen roses or to have roses around your home and workplace. They will attract love to you. It is also helpful to eat rose sweets or rose-flavoured Turkish delight, and to share them with both friends and potential sweethearts.

∽ **Rose for marriage.** Perform the Somerset love spell. Pluck and use the white rose as outlined above.

∽ **Rosehips for personal protection, or for a child blessing.** Collect rose hips and string them into a necklace. Wear it for psychic protection. You can make one for yourself, for a friend, or for a child. We recommend using green thread to string the rosehips on; green is the colour of the love goddess Venus and the colour of love.

∽ **Rose for secrets to be kept.** For privacy and discretion about things spoken, put roses above head height or hang them from the ceiling. If you are hosting a confidential meeting or a secret get-together, having roses hung above you is an effective magical method to stop word getting out and prevent rumours starting.

Rosemary

Rosemarinus officinalis. Attribution: Sun (Culpeper and Lilly) Rosemary, that aromatic herb we know as a seasoning in cooking, is one of the most powerful magical plants of all. It is used in many hundreds of charms, spells and customs. Rosemary emanates the power of dominion, rulership; Robert Hacket's 1607 wedding sermon expresses it succinctly:

Rosemary ... which by name, nature and continued use, man challengeth as properly belonging to himself. It overtoppeth all the flowers in the garden, boasting man's rule. Another property of the Rosemary is, it affecteth the hart. Let this Rosmarinus, this flower o' men, insigne of your wisdom, love and loyaltie, be carried not only in your hands, but in your heads and harts.

This passage in the sermon alludes to the fact that men held sprigs of rosemary and wore them in weddings. [319] This was because they were to be rulers over their wives in the marriage to come. But even back then it was understood that this power could belong to women. There is a saying, 'Where Rosemary flourishes, the lady rules.'[320] Some say it will only grow in the garden of a house ruled by a woman; others say it will grow only for a good woman.[321] Rosemary's association with women goes way back. In ancient Greece, rosemary played a part in the cult of Aphrodite/Venus.[322] Since the Middle Ages, it has been given to the Virgin Mary (it is literally the 'rose of Mary').

In southern England, rosemary is above all a plant of friendship—Hampshire people used to call it 'the friendship bush'. People in London plant a rosemary bush in their garden if they want to attract friends. A Spanish proverb says rosemary is a plant of love.[323] Thomas More wrote, 'it is the herb sacred to remembrance and therefore to friendship'.[324] Rosemary conjures remembrance, whether of a friendship or other memories. Famous is the phrase 'rosemary for remembrance' (Ophelia in *Hamlet*). An old folk custom for curing bad dreams is to put rosemary under the sleeper's bed.[325] But it is not only a cure for bad dreams but a herb to help the sleeper have visionary dreams, as this elaborate spell outlines.

Three Women's Prophetic Dream Working
This working for prophetic dreams must be done by three women under the age of twenty-one years on the eve of St Magdalene's Day (22 July).

Ingredients: rum, wine, gin, vinegar, three sprigs of rosemary
Equipment: a jar of ground glass, three pins
Place: upstairs bedroom, with a bed large enough for three
The three must go to an upper room of the house, i.e. a bedroom: in a vessel of ground glass, mix wine, rum, gin and vinegar. Into this mixture they must dip three sprigs of rosemary, and then pin the sprigs to their dress. After this each must take three sips of the mixture. Then all three must lie down in the same bed and go to sleep. The resultant dreams will be prophetic ones.[326]

Rosemary

It is unsurprising, given its great power, that rosemary is also used for protection. It is employed against supernatural attack and poltergeists, in particular attack by fairies and spirits.[327]

∽   **Rosemary for gaining authority.** Use rosemary to give a person authority in their relationships, including those in their work environment, for example, where a person needs to be respected as a boss or an expert but they are not receiving this respect. It is thus particularly useful for people of colour, for introverts, or for people on the autistic spectrum who have a dominion of expertise to share. If you give a bunch of rosemary to somebody, we recommend tying it with ribbons which are coloured red and purple, the colours of assertiveness and respected authority.

∽   **Rosemary for friendship.** Give a new friend a sprig of rosemary to help the friendship grow. Plant a friendship bush to attract friends; or give a friend who is moving to a new area a potted rosemary to plant so they attract new friends at their new home. Ideally, the pot should be green, or tied with a green ribbon, this being the colour which promotes friendship and affection.

∽   **Rosemary for remembrance.** Use rosemary where remembrance—emotional memory—is to be conjured. Use it for spells which conjure nostalgia and when you want someone to remember times from their past, or to recall old friendships. Wear a sprig to a funeral or a memorial service. Place a sprig in front of a photo of a departed or lost friend. If you want someone from your past to remember you, find an object or picture associated with your time together, place a sprig of rosemary on it and light a candle next to it.

∽   **Rosemary against nightmares.** Use rosemary in a spell against nightmares. We suggest making a little pillow or sachet and stitching rosemary and as many of the other anti-nightmare herbs you can locate into it. The pillow should be of the colour blue, the colour of the moon, who rules dreams and sleep.

∞   **Rosemary for women.** Use rosemary in spells to give a woman authority in her marriage or any relationship where it is a man who holds the most power. An easy way to do this is to give the woman a rosemary pot plant. If the woman needs authority at home, we suggest putting it on a kitchen windowsill; one can easily commune with the rosemary spirit while doing the washing up or making tea each morning. We recommend tying a purple ribbon around the pot, or colouring the pot itself. Purple is the colour of authority and honour.

∞   **Rosemary for protection.** Use rosemary especially for protection from attack by supernatural beings. This is experienced as a bad atmosphere or an unusually long run of bad luck and strange misfortunes. The most effective way to use rosemary in this instance is to put it on to incense charcoals so it smoulders and produces smoke. The whole home or affected area should be censed, and everyone affected should breathe in the scented smoke.

∞   **Rosemary for prophecy.** If you are a woman aged under twenty-one, you might perform the prophecy working outlined above with two friends.

Rowan

Also known as mountain ash, witchen tree, witchwood, quicken tree.

Sorbus aucuparia. Attribution: none in Culpeper or Lilly

The rowan is one of the most important plants of British folk magic. It is a common tree in the British Isles, found all over London's streets and parks, and it has distinctive orange-red berries which come out in August and September. Folklore says that rowan trees are the home of the 'light elves', (whatever these may be). One may see them by visiting a rowan, particularly at night, or on an old day of magic such as May Day Eve or Hallowe'en.[328]

But the rowan is famed for its astonishingly powerful ability to repel bad magic and misfortune. Its power is recognised across England, Ireland, Scotland, Germany and Sweden, and in the British Isles it was so universally prized that at Christian festivals rowan was sometimes given out by the clergy to the members of the congregation to preserve them from evil spirits. Its power is shown by its berries, for people say of the berries' redness, 'there is no better colour against the devil'.[329]

The rowan is exalted in song, poetry and story. One famed couplet runs, 'Rowan tree and red thread, hold the witches all in dread.'[330] The rowan also features in the ballad 'Laidley Wood':

> The spells were vain, the hag returned
> To the queen in sorrowful mood
> Crying that witches have no power
> Where there is row'n-tree wood.[331]

What do people use rowan to protect against? The answer is everything: people, work tools, animals, the home. Most commonly, the method is to tie or attach sprigs of rowan.[332] For many, it is customary to keep some in their pocket.[333] In Lancashire, rowan sprigs are hung at bed heads. In Cornwall and Somerset, farmers wind rowan around their cattle's horns.[334] In Scotland, the method is to make a cross of rowan with red thread; this is put anywhere that is to be protected, but often sprigs are put into the lining of the clothes. The Scottish also have the custom of making a ring of the twigs or berries, then passing the cherished object through the circlet; on a grander scale, large hoops can be made from branches and livestock passed through them.[335] The power of the rowan to protect is sometimes called upon specifically against the evil eye, which is the ill luck caused by someone's envy or jealousy of you.[336]

Many people believe the best time to do rowan protection work is at sunset on May Eve.[337] May Eve (Beltane) is a prescribed time to protect things with rowan in Carmarthenshire in Wales and possibly more widely across Wales; and across Scotland.[338]

∞ **Rowan for protection.** Cut some twigs of about two or three inches long. Make small, equal-armed crosses with them, by binding the central joining point with red string or yarn. Wrap it around several times so they are secure. This is your simple protection cross. Make several, and hang them on the things you wish to protect from harm.

∞   **Rowan for protection (Scottish method).** Get some longer young branches of rowan and bend them into a hoop, ideally using red-coloured string or yarn. Then pass through the hoop those things you wish to be protected. You can do this at any time, but it is especially effective to do it at Beltane (the eve of May Day).

∞   **Rowan for seeing elves.** Visit the tree at night, or on May Eve, or on Hallowe'en. We recommend going at midnight.

Rue

Also known as herbgrace, herb-of-grace.
Ruta graveolens. Attribution: Sun (Culpeper), Saturn (Lilly)
Rue is a wild-flowering herb which gardeners nowadays sometimes employ as an ornamental plant. It is not to be underestimated, however. Rue is one of the two herbs most frequently mentioned as a plant of witches (the other is vervain) in southern England witch-trial records. An ingredient in the imagined potions of ill intent, it was thought to be one of the herbs witches stirred in their cauldrons deep in the night. Symbolically, rue stands for repentance, which seems contradictory, but it could be that people thought an evil witch used rue to make someone have regret for something they have done ('you'll be sorry, you'll see').

Rue is used in folk magic to stop yourself from doing something you would later regret. Perhaps unexpectedly, it is deemed good for mental health: Drayton's account of a witch's potion to cure insanity includes rue: 'Then sprinkles she the juice of Rue, with nine drops of the midnight dew, from Lunary distilling.'[339]

∞   **Rue for restraint.** Take a little of the herb rue with you wherever you go, in a small bag, and nibble some when you have the urge to undertake an action you'll regret. You will find that you are able to restrain your impulse. If you pick the rue yourself, speak to the spirit of the plant before plucking the twig, giving thanks and asking its blessing.

∞ **Rue for protection against the evil eye.** Use rue against the evil eye. What folklore calls the evil eye is the bad luck which comes from another person's jealousy being directed towards you. Herbs which are effective against the evil eye are the ones to use when you know that you have something which arouses other people's malicious envy. Use rue, then, to encircle and protect the thing which is the focus of this envy. So, if you are a dancer, it may be your dance shoes; if you are wealthy, your chequebook; if you are a homeowner, the periphery of your premises.

∞ **Rue for spiritual equilibrium and mental wellbeing.** This old remedy is one which involves advance planning. The potion requires preparation, as the method is to sprinkle rue juice with nine drops of midnight dew and distil with a bit of honesty (modern name of the herb lunary). First, buy or borrow and set up a wine-making kit. Read the instructions. Crush some fresh rue to extract the juice, then put this on a saucer. At midnight, go out and find leaves with dewdrops on, then shake nine drops on to the rue juice. Take it indoors and add some honesty herb, then use the herb mixture to make wine.

Saffron
See crocus

Sage
Salvia officinalis. Attribution: Jupiter (Culpeper), Saturn (Lilly) Mainly a medicinal plant found in every herbal pharmacy, sage is ruled by Jupiter.[340] It is a plant long associated with wisdom—hence the name 'sage'. Interestingly, it is folklorically linked with women as well. In the Cotswolds and possibly elsewhere, the sage bush is a feminine plant, one which flourishes where the woman dominates the household, that 'the mistress is master'; one folklore collector relates the case of a husband who chopped down a flourishing sage bush in his front garden lest the neighbours think his wife ruled the house.[341] It is also good for love; it is the central ingredient in an old love spell.

Old Sage Love Spell

Take three sage leaves. Write 'Adam, Eve' on the first leaf; write 'Jesus, Mary' on the second leaf, and write your own name on the third. Then grind the three leaves and put the powder into the drink or food of the person you love. When they have consumed it, in a very short time they will love you.[342]

∞ **Sage for women's power.** The woman who wishes to increase her authority should plant a sage bush near her home, or plant one in a pot as a houseplant. Attention and focus while doing so are important, and she should speak to the sage throughout. Once it is planted, she must tend it closely so it flourishes. We suggest putting the plant on a kitchen windowsill so it is handily placed; one can easily commune with the sage while doing the washing-up or making tea each morning. We recommend tying a purple ribbon around the sage pot or colouring the pot itself purple (the colour of authority and honour).

∞ **Sage for making a person love you.** Perform the Old Sage Love Spell above. We recommend avoiding doing love magic to make a person fall in love with you, because it involves another person's will.

Savory, summer

Satureia hortensis. Attribution: Mercury (Culpeper)

Summer savory is a common garden herb used in cooking. Its powers are those of arousing sexuality at its most wild, primal and driving. The ancient Greek writer Pliny wrote that satyrs, famously sexually rampant, lived in meadows of savory and ate a diet of savory. Satyrs, for the Greeks, were mythical half-man, half-goat beings who frolicked across the hills, loving enthusiastically and indiscriminately.

∞ **Summer savory for sex.** Use savory in a magical spell with the aim of inciting wild sexuality and ecstasy of the body and spirit. One option is to make a simple herbal tea of savory as part of a seduction evening. Alternatively, put a little bit of boiled savory water into some wine or juice. When working with the savory plant spirit, we recommend using cups or glasses or dishes which are red and green; these are the colours which vibrate on the frequencies of passion and love (Mars and Venus).

Saxifrage (Burnet saxifrage)

Also known as breakstone
Pimpinella saxifrage. Attribution: Moon (Culpeper)
This is a garden plant with tiny flowers. As a magical herb, it is often overlooked, but its powers are worth remembering. People use saxifrage to see witches; on the night before May Day (Beltane), people used to go outside and hold it tightly in their hands in order to see the witches, who were of course out and about that night. Also, it is cited as granting protection against evil forces in accounts from all over the British Isles, including Scotland.³⁴³ Saxifrage is also a beauty remedy: collecting fresh saxifrage and eating it makes one more attractive within days, it is claimed.³⁴⁴

∞ **Saxifrage to see supernatural witches.** On May Eve (Beltane), go outside with a bunch of saxifrage in your hand, and you will see the witches clearly. We recommend going out as far as you can into the wildest part of your neighbourhood, ideally to a copse of trees under which there is a shady enclosure.

∞ **Saxifrage for attractiveness.** First, find fresh saxifrage, then eat some—either raw or cooked. You will become visibly more attractive within a day or two. We recommend speaking kindly to the plant spirit beforehand and eating or drinking the herb from a dish or cup which is green in colour—green is the colour of Venus, so in magic, it is understood that the things of the colour green emanate love and beauty.

Self-heal

Prunella vulgaris. Attribution: Venus (Culpeper)
This is a wild countryside plant which is rarely used in folk magic. However, the one mention we did find is a good one. In Hampshire, they say that if you go out picking self-heal, the devil will come and carry you away.³⁴⁵

✐ **Self-heal to visit fairy realms.** To be taken away to supernatural realms, possibly even by the 'devil', go out and pick self-heal. To do this, first learn to identify the plant, then go out in your local area and find a patch where it grows. Once you've done that, you can plan an outing to go self-heal gathering. We recommend organising your outing to take place on the night of a full moon. Even better is to do it on a night when the fairies are known to be out and about (May Eve, Midsummer's Eve, Lammas Eve, or Hallowe'en). We also suggest you take an offering for the fairies and place it in the midst of the plant patch: traditional offerings include milk, cream or whiskey.

Sesame

Genus *Sesamum.* Attribution: none in Culpeper or Lilly

Sesame is a plant with tiny white seeds which are used in cooking, most commonly on burger buns; you can buy small packets of them from most supermarkets. Sesame seeds have the power to open the ways into the caves of mountainsides or underground caverns, as well as doors. This lore comes from Arab culture, and it is from there that we get the phrase, 'Open, sesame!'[346]

✐ **Sesame for opening doors and for gaining access to closed spaces.** Take a small handful of sesame seeds to the door or gate that is locked. We recommend carrying them in a box or fabric carrier of mixed colours, as mixed colours have the power of Mercury, god of tricksome solutions. Mercury's powers are the powers of pickpockets, thieves and quick, unlikely changes. As for timing, we recommend doing this at midnight. Once you are in front of the locked door, stand firmly and sprinkle the seeds, then speak or sing to gain the assistance of the sesame plant spirit. You can also use sesame to unblock your access to a place you wish to enter, for example, a university, an art school or an invitation-only meeting.

✐ **Sesame for opening mountain caves.** As above, sprinkle the seeds, singing or speaking to ask for the assistance of the sesame spirit. This will be useful for people working with mines and mining, or who are digging tunnels, including train tunnels and similar.

St John's wort

Hypericum Perforatum. Attribution: Sun (Culpeper and Lilly) This plant has small, delicate yellow flowers and perforated leaves; the extracted oil has a distinctive red colour. St John's wort is one of the most important plants of all in European folk magic, and its leading power is protection. The plant is named hundreds of times in old recipe books, poems, charms and rhymes. It scares away bad beings: 'St John's Wort, scaring from the midnight heath, the witch and goblin with its spicy breath.'[347] Another name for it is *fuga daemonum* (devil's flight).[348] Here is what is said in one old poem of a lady who was guarding a man in her house from demonic attack:

> St John's Wort and fresh Cyclamen she in her chamber kept
> From the power of evil angels to guard him while he slept.'[349]

The devil or his demons cannot be in the same room as a person wearing sprigs of the herb. The devil says to one seeker, 'Gin you would be leman of mine, lay aside the St John's Wort and the Vervain' ('If you would be a true love of mine, throw away your St John's wort and vervain.')[350]

St John's wort is a herb that is traditionally gathered on St John's Eve, or Midsummer's Eve.[351] John Stow, in his *Survey of London*, relates that Londoners of his day would have St John's wort all around their house at midsummer. Hung up at doors and windows that same day, it drives away demons and evil powers from the home as the nights start to grow longer.[352]

Being a plant of the sun, it brings not only light to banish the dark (demons), but also the solar blessings of health and happiness. If you cannot wait till midsummer for your magical working, you can follow the instructions of the old remedy which promises that the herb will cure a person's melancholy 'if it is gathered on a Friday in the hour of Jupiter, and worn away about the neck'.[353] Scotland, in particular, is a place where a bit of the plant is worn as an amulet.[354] In England, some believe that placing some of the herb in a shoe will keep a traveller from tiring.[355] From the Scottish Western Isles comes this charm, which you should say when you pick St John's wort:

> St John's wort, St John's wort,
> You are envied by whoever has you.
> I will pluck you with my right hand,
> I will carry you in my left hand.
> Whoever finds you in their cow-barn,
> Will never be without cattle.[356]

∾ **St John's wort for house protection and home happiness.** St John's wort flowers in June and July, so this is the time to gather the plant. Use the sprigs or branches to decorate above your doorways and put some sprigs in vases around your home. It is of course traditional to do this on Midsummer's Day, but if that's not possible, you can do it any time. If it is not the right season, or you don't have plants growing locally, you can use the dried herb, which you can buy from a shop or online. However or whenever you get the herb, we advise using gold or yellow ribbon or fabric to wrap it; gold is the colour of the sun, the colour which emanates health, wealth and wellness in harmony with the powers of St John's wort itself.

∾ **St John's wort for travel energy, and for long-distance running.** Put some of the herb in the sole of your shoe so that you do not tire when going by foot. A tiny sprig of the plant makes a nice gift for a friend who is going away on a journey that will require some physical effort, such as visiting Macchu Picchu or climbing in the mountains. We recommend drying a few small leaves flat between the pages of a book before the date of the friend's departure. Then slip the flat, dried leaves into a card. They can put them into their shoes if they wish. This gift is also appropriate for a friend who is a long-distance runner; no matter how far they have to run, they will not tire.

∞ **St John's wort for happiness, against melancholy.** If you do have the plant growing near you and you want to get some at a time other than midsummer, gather it on a Friday. To use the plant's powers for personal protection, wear it around your neck. You can do this by putting some into a small charm bag, ideally one made of yellow cloth, or alternatively put it into a gold locket, using a string or chain to make it into a necklace.

∞ **St John's wort for personal protection.** Keep some leaves and flowers of the plant near you or on you. Wear some around your neck in the form of an amulet. As mentioned above, it is easy to make a small charm bag, ideally from yellow cloth. If you have a gold locket, you can put the St John's wort into it and clasp it closed. Hang it on a necklace or a string around your neck.

St John's blood

St John's wort oil is called St John's blood.

This gruesomely named liquid is simply the oil of St John's wort, which has a distinctive red colour. The oil is best if it is from plants gathered on Midsummer's Day, and some people specify that the plants should be picked at midnight.[357] St John's blood is highly effective against curses and demonic attacks. This has been its main use for hundreds of years, but people have used it for other purposes, too. In Germany, people rub it on the barrels of their guns so their shots will hit their targets. Others rub it on their clothes to have success in gambling. The oil is especially popular in Dutch and Germanic areas, and in Sicily, where healing powers are attributed to it.[358]

∞ **St John's blood for luck in gambling.** Once you have made the oil, use it on yourself as you prepare for an event in which you will be taking chances. This could be playing games of chance, but equally it could also be when you are about to take a big gamble. Perhaps you're bidding in an auction, buying something sight unseen, taking a risk in your personal life, or taking a gamble in business. As you get dressed, use it lightly on your skin. Then put a small drop on the things you will be using: maybe dice, maybe cards, but maybe on your phone, laptop or relevant documents.

∽ **St John's blood for hitting targets.** Rub on the barrel of your gun or bow, before shooting.

∽ **St John's blood for personal protection.** Anoint yourself with some of the oil as you get ready to face the wider world, or a situation in which you feel you need protection from bad energies or ill fortune.

Thistle, Scotch
Also known as cotton thistle, woollen thistle, down thistle
Onopordum acanthium. Attribution: Mars (Culpeper)
The Scotch thistle, the purple-spiked plant that is the emblem of Scotland, is only occasionally used in folk spells. One use, however, survives from the Mediterranean in the late antique period; this is to make a thistle amulet to give relief from feelings of worry and dread. Find when the moon will be in Capricorn, and at that time go out and pluck a Scotch thistle, then wear it or carry it with you. If you have this thistle on you, you will have peace of mind.[359]

∽ **Thistle for peace of mind, against anxiety.** Make a thistle amulet. This is best done in August or September: thistles flower between late July and early October. First, find where a thistle grows in your local area, then look up when the moon will next be in Capricorn, using an online moon-phase calculator. On that day, go out to your thistle plant, speak kindly to the thistle spirit, then cut the thistle flower. Take it home and make it into an amulet by encasing it in a small box. It will be too prickly to wear or carry if it is encased in fabric. We recommend using a box of purple and/or green in the box, as these are the colours of Jupiter (expansiveness, steady success) and Venus (love, growth, friendship). Wear or carry the thistle amulet as you go about your day.

Thyme

Thymus vulgaris. Attribution: Venus (Culpeper and Lilly)

Thyme is a well-known aromatic cooking herb especially popular in French cooking. In both the ancient world and medieval physic, it is sacred to Venus. In the Mediterranean, in Eryx, Sicily, people brought basketfuls of roses and thyme to her statue.[360] In terms of magical uses and powers, it is hugely important; its use in magic ranges across Europe and across centuries. In the medieval period and later, people believed that witches, fairies and elves love thyme, and so these supernatural creatures live in banks where its bushes grow. There are numerous examples of the lore, but the most famous is in Shakespeare's *A Midsummer Night's Dream*, where the fairy king Oberon says, 'I know a bank where the wild thyme blows.'[361]

As for the plant's specific powers, they are several. Foremost, it offers protection from evil and negative forces. To this end, people put it on their doors and windows, around the entrances to their barns, and so forth. It is a custom also to carry some thyme to protect you from disaster and to bring you good luck; in many areas, people (particularly young women) make and wear crowns of the herb for the same purpose.[362] In Germanic areas, thyme is hung up in the house to keep out witchcraft and bad spirits.[363]

Thyme is also a giver of courage: Roman soldiers put it into their baths to strengthen their resolve. In the Middle Ages, a lady would give a sprig of thyme to a knight errant for the same reason. Crusaders, too, wore thyme with courage in mind.[364]

∞ **Thyme for courage.** Have a thyme bath to fortify yourself. Simply take some fresh thyme, or a bit of dried thyme if you don't have access to fresh sprigs. In a little bowl, rub and crush it with a little oil; this helps release the scent. Put it into your warm bath and the scent will fill the bathroom as you bathe.

∞ **Thyme for space protection.** Hang it up in the house or around any area you wish to protect. Although there are many herbs which are good for protection, thyme is especially useful when you want the people in the space to be not only safe but brave. We recommend tying your bundles of thyme with red thread or string, as red is the colour of fortitude and lust. If you are sprinkling dried thyme around your house, we suggest dispensing it from a red bowl or a red cloth, for the same reason.

∾ **Thyme for personal protection.** For protection from harm and ill luck, carry some thyme in your pocket or bag. We recommend using thyme for protection in circumstances where you are facing conflict and need to be brave. In those circumstances, place it in a red bag or wrap. Thyme is sacred to Venus, so you can wear thyme in cases where you need the protection of the goddess of love; in those cases, surround the thyme with the colour green.

∾ **Thyme for contacting fairies.** Use thyme in rituals and spells to contact the fairy folk. A nice (and magical) summer activity is to go on a walk in your local area to find where the thyme grows wild, or in large amounts. If you can find a 'thyme bank'—that is to say, a grove of bushes—you have probably found a place where the fairies live. It is a nice thing to leave an offering. If you're not sure how to identify the plant, take a little culinary thyme with you to compare the scent of the crushed leaves with those on likely-looking bushes.

∾ **Thyme to honour Venus, goddess of love.** Have a plant in the house to honour Venus. It is the best to have, above all others, when you need courage in love. It brings courage, and at the same time is sacred to the goddess of love.

Valerian

Valeriana officinalis. Attribution: Mercury (Culpeper), Venus (Lilly)

Valerian is a plant of many and various magical powers, appearing in many charms and magical workings. Its reputation is deeply sorcerous, too. Chaucer says it is one of the herbs that magicians put into their potions:

> And herbes coud I tell eke many (much more) on
> As Egremain, Valerian and Lunarie
> ... to bring about our craft, if that we may

When dried, valerian smells strongly of old socks—not terribly pleasant. Smell notwithstanding, people swear by its occult potencies. Valerian has the power to give you friends in high places. An old charm recounts how it will endear you to royalty and those at court; it comforts the person who wants the love of lords and ladies, of kings and queens. It makes the unworthy worthy. It makes sad people happy. It makes the poor rich. It makes people get whatever they want.[365] Albertus Magnus says 'valeria' juice makes peace between people warring against one another.[366] It is also good for being popular romantically, as it has the power to inspire love.[367] In the west of England, people wear a sprig of valerian so as never to lack lovers.[368] One slightly more complex old valerian love spell survives, containing fragments of Catholic prayer, as was common in Protestant England.

Old English Valerian Love Spell
Gather valerian when the moon is in the south, saying the words, *Miserere mei beatus vir qui non intilliger* ('Have pity on me, a blessed man who does not understand'). Say three Pater Nosters, three Aves and the Creeds. Put the valerian under your tongue and kiss the person you love, and they will love you back.[369]

∾ **Valerian to gain influence.** Use valerian in spells to gain you friends and favours from people in positions of power, especially when your success depends upon connections and personal recommendations. This is often the case in the music business, the film industry, the theatre, and in start-ups.

∾ **Valerian to gain the love for a particular person.** Perform the old English spell above. Women should change the words *beatus vir* (blessed man) to *beata mulier* (blessed woman).

∾ **Valerian for truces and peacemaking.** To help end a quarrel, include valerian herb in your spells for peacemaking. You may include it in other ways, too. You might put a bouquet of flowers in the room of the truce meeting and have some valerian sprigs in the floral arrangements in the room.

∞   **Valerian for love.** Use valerian in love spells where charisma and popularity are desired; it is especially useful to do this when you are starting out on a phase of going on dates, as it helps you to become romantically appealing.

Vervain

Genus *Verbena*. Attribution: Venus (Culpeper), Venus and sometimes Saturn (Lilly)

Vervain is an extremely important magical herb in European folk magic, significant since as far back as ancient Greece. One name for it is enchanters' plant, and people have long believed that witches gathered it and used it in their nefarious conjurations. Witches and sorcerers 'used the plant in all sorts of magic recipes'.[370] Some, in fact, were scared to use this powerful plant in their charms or herbal medicine because it was so closely linked with witchcraft.[371]

If you want to gain magical powers, one of the oldest methods is to take vervain leaves, crush them, then rub your naked body with the leaves so the juice goes all over your skin and into your pores. This will give you incredible gifts: seeing the future, having your wishes come true, ending feuds with all your enemies, and complete protection from curses and psychic attacks.[372]

Paradoxically, it also gives protection *from* sorcery.[373] Since the Middle Ages, people have worn vervain against bad magic, and against the wiles of Satan, as it 'putteth aback devils'.[374] One late Roman herbal prescribed wearing a bit of it around one's neck to cure mental illness, which at the time was believed to be caused by negative forces.[375] Across Europe, vervain is hung up to keep out bad energies.[376] In early modern England, people would put it together with dill, as the combination was effective in repelling bad magic: as John Aubrey related, a rhyme of the time ran, 'Vervain and dill, hinder witches of their will.'[377] It will keep you safe from thieves while you are travelling if you carry some with you.[378] It even has a blessing or blessed quality. Ben Jonson wrote, 'Bring your garlands, and with reverence place the Vervain on the altar.'

Vervain

There are many rules and customs associated with pluck-ing vervain. It should be dug or cut with an implement made of silver or gold.[379] The plant should be addressed politely when it is collected, and there are many surviving picking charms. In Lancashire, they say, 'Hallowed by thou, vervain, if thou growest on the ground.'[380] In Elizabethan England, some would say:

> All hail, thou holy herb, Vervain
> Growing on the ground
> On the Mount of Calvary
> There was thou found.
> Thou helpest many a grief,
> And staunchest many a wound.
> In the name of sweet Jesus,
> I take thee from the ground.[381]

It is a plant which is deemed to be Venusian, full of the essence and quality of love, and is a common ingredient in love spells across Europe. Here's one German magical spell to make someone love you: at sunset, roll some vervain in your hands, then shake the hand of the person you desire and they will fall in love with you.[382] In some parts of Germany up through the nineteenth century, a bride was presented a wreath of vervain, 'as if to put her under the protection of Venus the Victorious'.[383] One of the most widely used magical guides says it is 'of great strength in venereal pastimes, that is, the act of generation'.[384] In the ancient world, its Venusian quality was also put to the use of friendship, and it was used for creating amity and jollity. Pliny says that if a hall is sprinkled with vervain-infused water, those who gather will be 'very pleasant and make merry more jocundly'.[385] It was used in wartime peace talks; Roman ambassadors would wear vervain crowns when going to meet enemies to negotiate war terms and treaties.[386] It is a herb that makes a child happy, as well as successful in learning: 'infants bearing it shall be very apt to learn, and loving learning, and they shall be glad and joyous'.[387]

The Greeks, the French and the English wear vervain as an amulet for health. A nineteenth-century folklore collector, one Mr Conway, reported seeing children with vervain tied around their necks as a luck and health amulet: he noted that people would wear a bit of vervain root tied with a length of white satin ribbon until they got better. Vervain is also good for financial health: 'If any man put it in his house or vineyard, or in the ground, he shall have abundantly revenues, or yearly profits.'[388] It is one of the herbs which, if prepared correctly, has the power to open locks. Make a small cut in your hand with a knife or scalpel; place a tiny bit of vervain on it and allow it to heal; after this, at your merest touch, 'keys would turn and bolts would slide'.[389]

∞ **Vervain for opening locks.** Perform the working outlined above.

∞ **Vervain for wellbeing.** Make a necklace of vervain, tying bits of the herb together with a nice ribbon. The colour of ribbon is not specified in the old lore, but it is commonly known that the best colour for health and wellbeing is gold, so we recommend making your necklace using a ribbon of a yellowy-gold colour.

∞ **Vervain for magical powers and psychic abilities.** Create a ritual which involves rubbing your skin with vervain juice. We recommend first crushing the vervain leaves and stems, with ceremony and with a rhyme or song. Remember that you are asking the blessing of the plant spirit to use it.

∞ **Vervain to make a wish come true.** Perform the ritual above.

∞ **Vervain for wealth.** Put the plant, or bunches of the herb, around your place of wealth generation—office, shop, computer, farmlands, etc. If you are tying the bunches with twine or ribbon, we recommend using some that is yellow or gold-coloured.

∞ **Vervain against thieves (during travel).** While travelling, put a sachet of vervain in your luggage and carry some on you in your purse. A traveller's 'good luck pouch' is a nice gift to make for a friend who is going on a journey.

Vervain

ൟ   **Vervain for peacemaking and truces.** Wear vervain
when entering arbitration, peace talks, or into a difficult conversation that you want to end peacefully. One option is to
rub vervain juice into your skin as part of the working. If you
are making a vervain sachet to wear during the talks, we recommend using a green bag. If tying a small bunch of vervain,
use a green ribbon. Green is the colour of Venus, goddess of
love and friendship.

ൟ   **Vervain for a baby or child blessing.** Use it in a child
blessing with the aim of making the child both happy and
clever.

ൟ   **Vervain for blessing relationships.** Wear vervain in a
crown, or find some other way to put yourself 'under' the
vervain. Perhaps put it over your bed, or wherever you spend
the most time with your partner. If tying the vervain, use a
green ribbon or twine, as green has the energy of Venus,
goddess of love.

ൟ   **Vervain for love spells.** Use vervain in love and erotic
magic spells. To make a person desire you, consider the
German handshake method above.

ൟ   **Vervain for protection.** Mix vervain with some dill, and
place the two herbs together on your person. Alternatively, put
them in the place where the ill-wishing is occurring, perhaps
your home or workplace. Vervain can also be used on its own:
put pinches of the dried herb around you, or fresh bunches
around your home.

ൟ   **Vervain for good parties and joyful gatherings.**
Sprinkle vervain water throughout the party space or venue.

Walnut tree

Genus *Juglans*. Attribution: Sun (Culpeper). Tree given to
Mercury but the nut to Venus (Lilly).
The walnut is a tree of foreboding power, to be treated
carefully. Among Greeks and Romans, it was the tree of
Persephone.[390] Across most of Europe, the lore of the walnut

128

tree is consistently negative; some believe that even its shade can make a person unwell. In Somerset, it is called 'the Devil's tree'.[391] In Italian lore, the walnut tree is known to be the residence of demons and the meeting place of witches; in fact, Italians call it 'the witch-tree'. Tuscany locals of the nineteenth century told a researcher, one Professor Giuliani, that 'witches love walnut trees'. Bologna folk said they knew that witches gathered at a walnut tree on midsummer. There is a famous demon-inhabited walnut tree in Benevento, uprooted by St Barbatus: but the spot where it was uprooted remains a meeting place for witches, and when they are about to gather, a walnut tree suddenly appears as if by magic on that same spot: as lush and large as the original.[392] One Benevento informant reported that 'as you walk beneath it of an evening, you may hear the servants of the devil whispering, snickering, and gibbering in its branches'.[393] Moving northwards to Germany, one finds that there, the black walnut tree in particular is a tree of evil, of ill fortune; this is in contrast with the oak, the tree emblematic of good fortune. And its worrisome reputation reaches as far as England, for in Somerset, the walnut 'is thought to be an evil tree'.[394]

Though the tree is dangerous, the nut is the friend to all. Walnuts are strewn at weddings as bringers of fertility to the couple.[395] People carry them to deflect and repel any spells that have been worked against them.[396] Some also use a walnut to see if someone has been doing magic against them, in this chair trick: put a walnut beneath the seat of a person suspected of sending psychic attacks; if they are issuing a curse, they will not be able to get out of the chair. If they can get up, then they are not using black magic.[397]

∽ **Walnut tree for meeting fairies.** Find a walnut tree local to you. Make a special pilgrimage to go and spend time sitting beneath it, mentally preparing yourself to meet supernatural witches and spirits. Midsummer's Day is a particularly good day for this.

∽ **Walnuts to repel spells done against you.** Bless or charge two walnuts, then put them in your pockets and carry them with you as you go about your day.

∞   **Walnut to discern an enemy.** Perform the chair trick above.

White bryony
See bryony, white

Willow
Also known as salley or sallow
Genus *Salix*. Attribution: Moon (Culpeper), Saturn (Lilly)
Willow trees are famed for growing by water, and one type, the iconic weeping willow, has long, slim branches which fall downwards to create a sheltering tent of foliage. Christian lore says Christ and his Apostles were met under a willow on the night of Jesus's agony, and the tree has wept ever since.[398] Italian lore says the weeping willow's leaves grow down because of the weight of angels' tears upon them; the angels are sorrowing for Adam and Eve's expulsion from the Garden of Eden.[399] Thus, it is no surprise that in magic and custom the willow is the tree sacred to the heartbroken and to dead loves. The willow as the tree of death goes back to ancient times: Circe has a grove of willows with hanging bodies; Persephone has a grove of willows and black poplars; Orpheus carries a willow branch in the underworld.[400] More recently, in England, Chatterton's song runs,

> Mie love ys dedde
> Gone to his death-bedde
> Al under the Wyllowe-tree.

The willow is not just for the bereaved lover but also for the rejected one. Spenser writes that the willow is 'worn of forlorn paramours'. A seventeenth-century English writer called it 'a sad tree, whereof such as have lost their love make their mourning garlands'.[401] An Irish folksong contains the lines from the mouth of the bereft lover:

> All around my hat
> I shall wear the green willow
> All around my hat
> for a twelvemonth and a day.

130

To send someone a willow garland signals a break-up, a tradition we see in Robert Herrick's poem, where one rejected lover writes of receiving one:

> A Willow garland thou did'st send
> Perfumed, last day, to me,
> Which did but only this portend—
> I was forsook by thee.

The tree is a supernatural one, a belief recognised across Europe, with local variants. The Irish say the willow has a soul which speaks in music; the Poles say the devil lives in it, and if you sit under a willow and renounce your baptism he will appear to you and give you psychic powers.[402] There and in other places, people report that strange and supernatural things happen to people when they are under the willow's branches.[403] Perhaps it is the devilish powers attributed to the willow which feed into the German use of the willow to slay distant enemies remotely by tying knots in a withie.[404] The spirit of the willow is recognised also in England, where people of the West Country believe that the tree goes walking at night, hauntingly following travellers in the dark. An old Somerset rhyme on the personalities of trees succinctly illustrates it:

> Ellum [elm] do grieve,
> Oak he do hate
> Willow do walk,
> If you travels late.[405]

Two catkin-laden willow branches feature in a Sussex spell to summon fairies. In the early twentieth century, an eyewitness reported the following, which had been done by Mrs Jasper, his nanny, when he was a child:

> You had to do it on a moonlight night when the pollen was just ripe on the [willow] catkins . . . She stood a few yards away [in a woodland clearing] with two small branches in her hands. I saw the gold dust flying from the catkins as she waved them gently, and she sang a little song over and

131

over in a low drawlin' husky voice—just as though she was coaxin' 'em:

Come in the stillness, Come in the night;
Come soon, And bring delight.
Beckoning, beckoning, Left hand and right;
Come *now*, Ah, come tonight![406]

∞ **Willow for healing heartbreak.** Find a nearby willow tree and spend time under it, meditating and contemplating: the tree is a comforter spirit. Wear a withie of willow around your hat, or some in your clothes. Doing so will help ease the emotional pain.

∞ **Willow for comfort in bereavement.** Find a willow tree near to your home, and spend time under it, meditating and contemplating: the tree is a comforter spirit. Wear a withie of willow around your hat, or some in your clothes. Doing so will help ease the emotional pain.

∞ **Willow for destroying distant enemies.** Employ the German technique of tying knots in a withie.

∞ **Willow for seeing fairies.** Perform the Sussex spell above.

∞ **Willow for ending a relationship.** Use willow leaves in your workings to help finalise the ending of a relationship. Willow is particularly appropriate to use when the partner you are leaving is having a hard time letting go.

Woodruff

Galium odoratum or *Asperula odorata*. Attribution: Venus (Culpeper)[407]

This aromatic herb grows across Europe, and everyone knows it to be a plant which evil witches fear. If you carry it on you, bad influences will stay away from you, so in several regions there is a long tradition of people carrying little bundles of it for protection. In Germanic areas, it is particularly common to use it for protecting babies and children; a bit of it is hung over a baby's bed or cradle for this purpose. Hanging a posy of woodruff over the bed of adults, too, keeps them well and blessed. As with many herbs, the spirit of the plant should be spoken to. Below is a Belgian charm which should be addressed to the woodruff spirit each night by a person who is using it for health and wellbeing:

> Blessed be, O holy herb,
> Make us healthy.
> First discovered on the Mount of Olives,
> You are good for so many woes,
> And heal so many wounds.
> Through the Lady's holy bouquet,
> Make us healthy, one and all.[408]

Woodruff extract is believed to give a person strength. In Germanic regions, around May time, a woodruff drink is prepared for everyone, to give them strength through the coming year. A modern version of this could be a home-made woodruff beer or wine, or a herbal tea.[409] English herbalist Nicholas Culpeper viewed it as a type of lady's bedstraw, and gave it the attribution of Venus, saying woodruff has the power of 'strengthening the parts ... which she [Venus] rules'.

∞ **Woodruff for protection.** Hang a small bouquet (a posy) of woodruff flowers over your bed, or, equally good, a sachet of the dried herb.

∞ **Woodruff for a baby blessing.** Include woodruff in a bag of blessing herbs to give to parents to hang near their baby's cradle.

∞ **Woodruff for inner strength.** Brew a woodruff beer, or make a wine or herbal tea of woodruff. Drink it, ideally around May Day.

Wormwood
Artemisia absinthium. Attribution: Mars (Culpeper)
The bitter wormwood, a small shrub with a strong aromatic scent, is little used in folk magic, except in England's West

Country. In Somerset, it is used against the evil eye.[410] In Devon, it is used against psychic attack.[411] There is an old custom to bring yourself good fortune through the whole of the coming year; it is done at midsummer, and it is simply to make a wormwood wreath, then throw it into the midsummer bonfire. In Italy, people make a girdle of wormwood to protect themselves while travelling, and in modern times drivers have updated the practice to hang a bundle of the herb in their car.[412]

∞ **Wormwood for protection during travel.** For a person who is going on a trip, a safe-travel bundle of wormwood makes a nice going-away present. The small bundle should be tied with orange ribbon, as that is the colour of travel, and done on a Wednesday. Equally, if you have recently acquired a car, you can bless its safety by washing it with warm water into which you have put a handful of wormwood. The old-fashioned method is to make a belt of wormwood, but this may be impractical in today's world.

∞ **Wormwood for good fortune through the year (midsummer).** On midsummer, it is a very lovely practice to make a wreath of wormwood as part of the celebrations. Making a bonfire is an old custom for this day. If you do this, too, you can continue with the old ritual and throw your wreath on to the fire at the end of the day.

Yarrow
Also known as milfoil, devil's nettle, mother-die
Achillea millefolium. Attribution: Venus (Culpeper)
Yarrow is a common British wildflower with flat-topped flower-heads which sit atop tough stems. It is sacred to Venus, goddess of love and friendship; this is attested by both the old herbals and by the folklore.[413] One charm for picking it runs, 'The pretty herb of Venus' tree/Thy true name it is yarrow.'[414] Yarrow has the power to attract old friends one wants to meet again. It draws distant people one seeks to connect with. 'It is a lucky weed to draw the attention of those you wish to see most.'[415]

Yarrow is used in divination, particularly in matters of love. The spell below is from old Scottish reports which say using yarrow was popular with young women, who would go out to 'cut it by moonlight with a black-handled knife', then employ it in a divination ceremony to foretell the future.

Scottish Yarrow Divination Spell

Find some yarrow growing in your area, noting the location; then go back on a moonlit night with a black-handled knife. Cut some sprigs of the yarrow with this knife, then use them in a ceremony of divination, to find answers to questions you have.[416] In the Scottish Hebrides, they say that you hold the yarrow's leaf against your eyes for a time; after this you will have what they call 'second sight'.[417] Perhaps the ceremony involved putting leaves against the eyelids.

English lore also offers yarrow spells to make you dream the future. Yarrow used to be abundant in graveyards, and people knew to pick yarrow, ideally from a graveyard, using words to address it as a living being.[418] It should be plucked at midnight or under a full moon, if the example of an old Devon spell is to be followed. Reported in the 1920s, the spell is as follows.

The South Devon Yarrow Divination Spell

If you want to dream of love for a man, you should first go to the graveyard. Then scout around until you find a young man's grave on which yarrow is growing. Make a note of its location, then go back there so that you will be there at midnight to pick it. Then, standing at the grave, at the point of midnight, address the yarrow plant growing on the grave thus:

Yarrow, yarrow, I seek thee, yarrow;
and now I have thee found.
I pray to the good Lord Jesus,
as I pluck thee from the ground.

Pull a stalk of the yarrow, and take it home. Get ready for bed, and as the last thing, put one sprig of the yarrow in your right sock; tie a second sprig to your left leg. Then get into bed backwards, saying:

135

Yarrow

> Good night to thee, yarrow.
> Good night to thee, yarrow.
> Good night to thee, yarrow.
> Once in bed you should say,
> Good night, pretty yarrow.
> I pray thee, sweet yarrow,
> tell me by the morrow,
> [here say what you want to know].[419]

If you want to dream of a woman, then accordingly, by deduction, you should find a young woman's grave which grows yarrow; and likewise the grave of whatever sort [of] person most appropriate for your particular question: the grave of a judge for legal matters, the grave of a suffragette for women's rights, etc.

Some say yarrow belongs to the Devil; it is sometimes known as devil's nettle.[420] But like many herbs feared for their power, it is also used for protection. In some regions, it is used to protect babies from evil supernatural witches: the adult ties a bit of yarrow to the cradle. For their own protection, the adult keeps a little yarrow in their pockets, or strews a bit on the threshold of their home.[421]

∽ **Yarrow to reconnect with an old friend.** Create a charm using a bit of yarrow, together with a picture of the person you wish to find again. If you don't own a picture, you can use anything they owned or something that has a connection to them. Put the charm in the place you think they will turn up—by your computer, if you're trying to connect online, or at work if they might come there, and so on.

∽ **Yarrow for getting an answer to a question in a dream.** Perform the South Devon Divination Spell above.

∽ **Yarrow for clairvoyance and psychic insight.** Devise a ceremony based around the Scottish Yarrow Divination Spell above. It should include blessing the yarrow and asking its help, then placing it on your eyelids.

∞   **Yarrow for personal protection.** Make a small twist or bag of yarrow and carry it on you, either in a bag around your neck, in your pocket, or even sewn into the lining of your jacket.

∞   **Yarrow for space protection.** Sprinkle some yarrow around the area you are protecting, remembering also to put a some on the threshold.

∞   **Yarrow for a baby blessing.** Tie a small bunch of yarrow with a ribbon. Give the posy to the parents to hang near the baby's cradle.

Yew

Taxus baccata. Attribution: Saturn (Culpeper and Lilly)

The dark and foreboding yew grows in graveyards and is known universally as a tree of doom and death. In the English Fens, people believe that witches live under the dark, drooping branches, so one should not spend time under the yew, lest one meet eerie supernatural beings.[422]

Since the tree can live for over a thousand years and is an evergreen, it is considered a tree of eternal life. The yew's powers of protection are especially used in Germanic areas. There, people would take a small piece of yew wood and tie it around their neck as an amulet for protection from evil magic. People also often make small, equal-armed crosses from yew twigs and hang them up in their storehouses, homes and barns. In some parts of Sweden, people would hang up entire yew branches for the same purpose: protection from bad witchcraft. Some would put the yew-twig crosses into their clothes, or tie them to their animals.[423] In the north of England, people use a yew twig to find lost objects; carrying it around, one will notice it twitch or jump when it is near the object lost, thus one can find it by searching further at that spot.[424]

∞   **Yew for space protection.** Put up branches of yew over the windows or doors, or in the rafters of the building you are protecting. Alternatively, take small twigs and from them make equal-armed crosses, tied with thread. Hang these up.

Yew

∞   **Yew for personal protection.** Make small, equal-armed crosses by tying two twigs with a thread or string. Put these in your pocket or the lining of your clothes or coat.

∞   **Yew for finding lost objects.** Get a yew twig, hold it in your hand and walk around the areas where you may have lost the item; it will twitch in your hand when you are close to what you have lost.

Spells and Potions
Using Multiple Herbs

Tyrolian Witch-viewer

Agrimony, broom, ground ivy, maiden-hair, rue

To see which women are witches, make a bundle of these five herbs. With this, you will know every woman for a witch who is one, no matter how unremarkable or unlike a witch she appears to you.[425]

Tyrolian Unbewitching

This is the method used by a Mr Kolb, one of Tyrol's first 'wonder doctors'. 'When he was called to assist any bewitched person, [he] made exactly at midnight the smoke of five different sorts of herbs, and while they were burning the bewitched person was gently beaten with a martyr-thorn birch, which had to be got the same night. The beating of the patient with the thorn was thought to be really beating the hag who had caused the evil.'[426]

To Hit a Target

Rue, vervain

In hunting or shooting, this magical technique will make your shot reach your aim: boil your gun-flints in a mixture of rue and vervain.[427]

To See Fairies

Hazel buds, hollyhock, marigold, thyme. Also grass of a fairy throne, marigold water, rosewater and salad oil

A seventeenth-century text in the Ashmolean contains this spell to see fairies.

141

A pint of sallat oyle put into a vial glasses: first wash it with Rose-water and Marygolde water: the flowers to be gathered toward the east. Warm it till the oyle becomes white. Then put it in the glasse, then put thereto the buds of Hollyhocke, the flowers of Marygolde, the flowers of wild Thyme, the buds of young Hazle and the Thyme must be gathered near the side of a hill where the fairies used to be: and take the grass of a fairy throne then all these put into the oyle in the glass and sette it to dissolve three days in the sunne and then keep it for thy use.[428]

Exorcism Water

Ash, basil, mint valerian, periwinkle, rosemary, sage
Make an aspersoir (water for sprinkling), which is effective for banishing evil spirits, by mixing the herbs together, grinding them into a powder and adding water.[429]

St Luke's Prophecy Powder Spell

Marigold, marjoram, thyme, wormwood
To foresee the future in a dream, perform the following spell on the old saint's day of St Luke, which falls on 18 October. However, before this, in early October, collect the herbs above and dry them. Nowadays, you can buy all of these already dried from internet herbal suppliers, but it is even better to pick them fresh in your neighbourhood. Get some old sheets which you don't mind getting stained and, on 18 October, change your bedsheets and put on these old ones. By your bed, put a notebook and pen. The herbs (if picked yourself) should now be dried; take about a tablespoon of each one and make into a powder in a mortar and pestle, if you have one. If not, you can use a blender. Put the powder into a bowl and add some spoonfuls of honey and a little vinegar until the blend is the same thickness as skin cream. Before you go to bed, smear the paste on your body with these words: 'Saint Luke, Saint Luke be kind to me; in dreams let me the future see.' Climb into bed with the paste still smeared on your body. Sleep and dream. When you awaken, make notes in the notebook by your bed straight away, as dreams are

swiftly forgotten. This is a young women's spell, and this version is faithful to the original except for two words in the charm: I have substituted, 'my truelove' with 'the future', as most people nowadays are not so focussed on whom they will marry.[430]

Disastrous Imaginings
Nettle, yarrow
This spell will make the person 'sure from all fear and fantasy, or vision', 'sure' meaning secure. Simply hold the yarrow and nettle together in your hand.[431]

To Rekindle Love
Houseleek, periwinkle. Also earthworms
To make a couple love one another again, take dried periwinkle and dried earthworms, grind to a powder, then mix the powder with houseleek. Put this mixture into the couple's food, and they will fall in love again.[432]

Charles I Coronation Oil
Ambergris, cinnamon, civet, jasmine, musk, orange flowers, rose, sesame
Charles I, on his coronation in 1626, decided to commission a special pleasantly scented oil for the chrism (anointing oil); Elizabeth I had said the oil used in her time was greasy and unpleasant smelling, so Charles's oil included the fragrant ingredients above. The oil was consecrated and enough was made for several coronations. It was only for the coronation of George VI, in 1937, that a new batch finally had to be prepared.[433]

Against Slander
Bay leaves, marigold, a wolf's tooth
Gather marigolds during when the sun is in Leo (23 July–22 August). Wrap them in bay leaves, then add a wolf's tooth to complete the bundle. Once you have this bundle and are

carrying it, 'no man shall be able to have a word to speak against you, but only words of peace'.[434]

St Agnes's Prophetic Dream Spell
Rosemary, thyme
To foresee the future in a dream, perform this spell on the eve of St Agnes's Day, an important night for workings of divination, dreams and prophecy. The eve is the night of 20 January. Before this, buy or obtain a sprig of thyme, and one of rosemary—these may well need to be dried specimens, as this date falls in the middle of winter. On the 20th, the Eve of St Agnes, think about the problem bothering you as you choose a pair of shoes to use for the spell. In one shoe, place a sprig of thyme and in the other some rosemary. Put a shoe on each side of the bed, and have a notebook ready to hand, then climb into bed, still thinking about whatever it is you are concerned about and feeling the presence of the herb-filled shoes on either side of your bed. Then say aloud, 'Saint Agnes that's to seekers kind, come ease the trouble of my mind.' Go to sleep, and on waking, make a note of your dreams in the notebook, quickly so you don't forget them. This spell is faithful to the original except for a single word in the charm: I have substituted 'lovers' with 'seekers', as what is concerning you may not be love.[435]

The Witch's Chain
Acorns, holly, juniper, mistletoe berries
This chain is made by three people, so they will be able to see the future. Make a chain of holly, juniper and mistletoe berries and place an acorn at the end of each link. Wind this chain around a long, thick log of wood. Performing magical rites, place it on the fire. As the last acorn is consumed by the flames, each person will have a vision of the future, and something will appear in the room which symbolises what is about to happen.[436]

To Believe Yourself a Witch

Centaury. Also bird blood (lapwing or black plover) and lamp oil

This spell will make someone believe they are a witch. Mix centaury with lapwing or black plover blood, then put this mixture into some lamp oil and light the lamp. All who gather round the lamp will think themselves witches: 'all they that compass it about shall believe themselves to be witches, so that one shall believe of another that his head is in heaven and his feet in the earth'.[437]

To Catch a Thief

Bay leaves, marigold, a wolf's tooth

Make the Against Slander bundle (above) and lay it under your head at night. In your dreams, you shall 'see the thief, and all his conditions'.[438]

To Create Disharmony

Peony seeds, vervain

This potion will create disharmony between two people. Gather vervain when the sun is in Aries (23 March–22 April). Gather peony seeds from a peony that is one year old. Dry both the vervain and the seeds, then grind them to a powder. Put the powder where the two people spend time together. 'If the powder be put in a place where men dwell, or lie between two lovers, anon there is made strife or malice between them.'[439]

Prophecy Perfume

Fleawort seeds, hemp seed, parsley, smallage (wild celery)

Make and wear this perfume if you wish to be able to see things to come, that is, to gain prophetic abilities. Mix the ingredients above, grind into a fine powder then make into a perfume using oil and alcohol.[440]

145

To Call the Fairy Sisters

Clove wood. Also ale, fair water, three new, white-handled knives and three white cloths

Plan ahead to meet the fairies and have a conversation with them: do this on the night before the new moon, or the night before the full moon. Stay up after everyone else in the house has gone to bed. All alone, then, sweep the hearth until it is very clean. Set out a bucket of fair water (clean fresh water) on the hearth. Go to bed. Be the first to get up the next morning; look for the fat or jelly which will have formed on the water in the bucket. Take it out with a silver or tin ladle or spoon, and set it aside. On the night before the new moon, or the night before the full moon, choose the room where you want to call the fairies, ideally one with an open fire, making sure that the house is silent and all is quiet, and on a table lay out:

> a bowl of new ale
> three new white cloths
> three new knives with white hafts

In the fireplace, make a fire of clove-wood. Sit in a chair facing the fire. Take the jelly and anoint your eyes with it. Sit silently and at rest. In due course, you will see three women come into the room. Say nothing to them, but do nod to them; they will nod back to you. They will go to the table and eat and drink, then file out of the room one by one. Let the first one pass by; likewise, the second; but when the third goes past you to leave the room, you may ask her any question you wish.[441]

Days and dates
for Magic

Monday	Tears, fluids, seas, wombs, dreams, visions, intuitions	Moon
Tuesday	Passion, assertiveness, aggression, ambitious drive	Mars
Wednesday	Quick messages, clear communication, gambling, good thinking	Mercury
Thursday	Long-lasting good fortune, endowment from institutions, benevolence from people in high places, personal maturity, the ability to be generous	Jupiter
Friday	Love, friendship, growth, springtime, pleasure, romance	Venus
Saturday	Refusals, endings, cut-offs, deadlines, death. Also earth matters: roots, caves, landownership, farming	Saturn
Sunday	Radiance, wellbeing, fame, confidence, recognition, sovereignty	Sun

Midwinter	Winter solstice, which falls around 20-22 December
Yule	Celebrated by pagans on winter solstice, by Christians on Christmas
New Year	Midnight of 31 December, though the end of the 1st of January
St Agnes Eve	Night of 20 January, leading to St Agnes Feast Day on 21 January
Imbolc	Night of 31 January through to sunset 1 February. Often conflated with Candlemas
Candlemas	2nd of February, Christian feast of the purification of the Virgin
Spring Equinox	Falls around 20-22 March
Beltane	Also called May Eve. Night of 30 April through sunset of 1st of May
May Day	1st of May
Midsummer's Eve.	The night before the summer solstice. Or, the night before St John's Day, thus the night of 23rd of June (some older European societies)
St John's Eve	Night of 23 June. Traditional beginning of midsummer in some societies
St John's Day	24 June. Traditional date marking midsummer in some societies
Lammas	Night of 30 July leading through to sunset of 1st of August
Autumn Equinox	Falls around 20-22 September
St Luke's Day	8th of October
Hallowe'en	Night of 31st of October
Samhain	Night of 31st of October through to sundown 1 November

Bibliography

Albertus Magnus [attrib.]. *The Book of Secrets of Albertus Magnus*, ed. Best and Brightman. Weiser, 1999.

Anon. 'The Four Leaves of the Truelove,' ed. and intro. Susanna Grier Fine. *In Moral Love Songs and Laments*. Medieval Institute Publications, 1998.

Anon. 'Herb Paris.' In *The Medieval Garden Enclosed: Metropolitan Museum Blog* [website]

Ayscough, Lady. *Lady Ayscough's Book of Receipts and Chirurgery* (1692). Reproduced by Charles Dickens in *Household Words V* (1852).

Coles, William. *The Art of Simpling* (1656). Kessinger, 2010.

Baker, Margaret. *Discovering the Folklore of Plants*. 3rd revised edn. Shire Publications, 2008.

Baker, Margaret. *Folklore and Customs of Rural England*. David & Charles, 1974.

Bane, Theresa. *Encyclopedia of Giants and Humanoids in Myth, Legend and Folklore*. McFarland, 2016.

Barber, Elizabeth. *The Dancing Goddesses: Folklore, Archaeology, and the Origins of European Dance*. Norton & Co., 2014.

Baose, Wendy. *The Folklore of Hampshire*. Batsford, 1976.

Bardswell, Frances. *The Herb Garden*. Adam & Charles Black, 1911.

Becker, Audrey, Kristin Noone and Donald Palumbo, eds. *Welsh Mythology and Folklore in Popular Culture: Essays on Adaptations*. McFarland, 2011.

Böhnert, K.-J. and G. Hahn. 'Phytotherapie in Gynäkologie und Geburtshilfe: vitex agnus-castus / Keuschlamm. Eine alte Kultur- un Arzneipflanze.' In *Erfahrungsheilkinde* 39 (1990), 494-52.

Bonser, Wilfred. 'Magical Practices against Elves.' In *Folklore* 37: 4 (31 December 1926), 350–63.

Brand, John. *Observations on the Popular Antiquities of Great Britain*. George Bell and Sons, 1877.

Briggs, Katherine. *The Folklore of the Cotswolds*. Batsford, 1974.

Burgess, Elizabeth. *Meadow Keep: Celebrating the History, Folklore and Superstitions of Herbs*. AuthorHouse, 2013.

Charnock, *Garden Spell: Magic of Herbs, Trees and Flowers*. Pavilion, 1994.

Culpeper, Nicholas. *Complete Herball* (1653). Ed. George Chapman and Marilynn Tweddle. Cambridge University Press, 1996.

Daniels, Cora Lyn and C. M. Stevans. *Encyclopedia of Superstitions, Folklore and the Occult Sciences of the World*. 2 vols. Yewdale & Sons, 1903.

Davies, Marion. *The Magical Lore of Herbs*. Capall Bann, 1994.

De Cleene, M. and Marie-Claire Lejeune. *Compendium of Symbolic and Ritual Plants in Europe*. Mens & Cultuur, 2003.

De Gubernatis, Angelo. *La Mythologie des plantes, ou Les Légendes du règne végétal*. Reinwald, 1882.

Dietz, S. Theresa. *Floriography Today: The Symbolic Meanings & Possible Powers of Trees, Plants and Flowers*. 2nd revised edn. Fayshoneshire, 2015.

Dyer, T. F. Thistleton. *The Folk-lore of Plants*. Hardwicke & Bogue, 1889.

Folkard, R. *Plant Lore, Legends and Lyrics*. Sampson, Low, 1892.

Friend, Hilderic. *Flower Lore*. Reprint of *Flowers and Flower Lore* (1884) with revised title. Para Research, 1981.

[Gauntlet, Arthur]. *Grimoire of Arthur Gauntlet*. Ed. D. Rankine. Avalonia, 2011.

Gordon, Lesley. *Green Magic*. Webb & Bowen, 1977.

Grieve, M. *A Modern Herbal*, 2 vols. Jonathan Cape, 1933.

Grigson, Sophie. *Sophie Grigson's Herbs*. BBC Books, 1998.

Hatfield, Gabrielle. *Hatfield's Herbal*. Allen Lane, 2007.

Harland, John, and Thomas Turner Wilkinson, *Lancashire Folk-lore* (1867). EP Publishing, 1973.

Howells, W. *Cambrian Superstitions*. Longman, 1831.

Johnston, John. *The Idea of Practical Physick in Twelve Books ... / written in Latin by John Johnston ...; and Englished by Nich. Culpeper, Gent. ... and W.R.* (1657).

King, R. J. 'Sacred Trees and Flowers', *Quarterly Review* (July 1863).

Knab, Sophie. *Polish Customs, Traditions and Folklore*. 2nd revised edn. Hippocrene Books, 1996.

Lansdell, Henry. *Through Siberia*. 2 vols. Sampson Low, 1882.

Lawton, Jocelyne. *Flowers & Fables: A Welsh Herbal*. Seren, 2006.

Le Sueur, F. *Flora of Jersey*. Société Jersiaise, 1984.

Lecouteux, Claude. *Traditional Magic Spells for Protection and Healing*. Inner Traditions, 2017.

Mac Coitir, Niall. *Irish Wild Plants: Myths, Legends and Folklore*. Collins, 2007.

MacLeod, Sharon. *Celtic Myth and Religion: A Study of Traditional Belief*. McFarland, 2011.

McCleery, Iona, et al. 'You are What You Ate'. School of History, University of Leeds [website].

Morrison, Melissa. *Dr Christopher's Herbal History* [website].

Northall, G. F. *English Folk Rhymes: A Collection of Traditional Verses Relating to Places and Persons, Customs, Superstitions, Etc*. Kegan Paul, 1892.

Northcote, Lady Rosalind. *The Book of Herbs*. 2nd edn. John Lane, 1912.

Navarra, Tova, and Myron Lipkowitz. *Encyclopedia of Vitamins, Minerals, and Supplements*. Facts on File, 2004.

Ovid, Fasti. Ed J. G. Frazer. *Fastorum libri sex: The Fasti of Ovid* (Cambridge Library Collection: Classics). Heinemann, 1931.

Palmer, Kingsley. *The Folklore of Somerset*. Batsford, 1976.

Palmer, Roy. *The Folklore of Warwickshire*. Batsford, 1976.

Percy, Thomas. *Reliques of English Poetry* (1765). Cambridge University Press, 2014.

Picton, Margaret. *Book of Magical Herbs: Herbal History, Mystery and Folklore*. Barron's Educational Series, 2000.

Piggott, H. 'Suffolk Superstitions'. *In The Gentleman's Library: Being the Classified Collection of the Chief Contents of The Gentleman's Magazine from 1731 to 1868—Popular Superstitions*. Elliot Stock, 1884, 122–32.

Reade, William Winwood. *The Veil of Isis, or The Mysteries of the Druids*. Skeet, 1861.

Rich, Vivian. *Cursing the Basil and Other Folklore of the Garden*. Heritage House, 2000.

Ryan, William. *The Bath House at Midnight: An Historical Survey of Magic and Divination in Russia*. Penn State, 1999.

Simpson, Jacqueline. *The Folklore of Sussex*. Batsford, 1973.

Skinner, Charles. *Myths and Legends of Flowers, Trees, Fruits, and Plants*. Lippincott Library, 1911.

Southwell, David, et al. *Hookland* [online community].

Thompson, Francis. *Supernatural Highlands*. Hale, 1976.

Teirlinck, Is. Flora magica: De plant in de tooverwereld. De Sikkel, 1930.

Tongue, R. L. *Somerset Folklore*. Folk-Lore Society, 1965.

Turner, William. *New Herball* (1551–68). Cambridge University Press, 1995.

Various. *The Customs, Beliefs, and Ceremonies of South Eastern Russia—The Khazar and Mordvin Kingdoms*. Pierides Press, 2010.

Verband Deutscher Vereine für Volkskunde. *Handwörterbuch des Deutschen Aberglaubens*. 10 vols. De Gruyter, 1927–42.

Vickery, Roy. *Dictionary of Plant-lore*. Oxford University Press: Oxford Reference, 1995.

Vickery, Roy. *Garlands, Conkers and Mother-Die*. Continuum, 2010.

Watts, D. C. *Dictionary of Plant Lore*. Academic, 2007.

Wright, Colin. *Artemisia*. Taylor and Francis, 2002.

Notes

1 Thompson, 97. Vickery, *Dictionary*, 1.
2 Gauntlet, 299. Folkard, 161.
3 Hatfield, 1.
4 Lecouteux, 109.
5 Baker, *Folklore of Plants*, 11.
6 Tongue, 31.
7 Hatfield, 4.
8 Friend, 32, with references on 628. De Cleene I:74.
9 Hatfield, 4.
10 Folkard, 209.
11 De Cleene, I:74.
12 De Cleene, I:74–5.
13 De Cleene II:40–42.
14 Skinner, 42. Folkard, 212.
15 Dyer, 62.
16 De Cleene II:42.
17 Folkard, 216.
18 Grieve, 36.
19 Folkard, 104. Brand III:16.
20 Vickery, *Dictionary*, 4.
21 Modern magical herbal writer Scott Cunningham gave it to Jupiter, which I would not follow. Culpeper attribution is implied.
22 Grieve, I:42.
23 Daniels and Stevans, II:873.
24 Daniels and Stevans, I:532.
25 Tongue, 176–7.
26 De Cleene, I:117.
27 De Cleene, I:117, citing Oomen.
28 De Cleene, I:117.
29 Friend, 302.
30 Dyer, 52.
31 Thompson, 97.
32 Baose, 139.
33 Baker, *Rural England*, 92.
34 Friend, 298.
35 Tongue, 166.
36 Brand, III:290, I:379.
37 Navarra, 133. Folkard, 246–7.
38 Morrison [online].
39 Folkard, 237.
40 Morrison [online].
41 De Cleene, II:56.
42 Rich, 12–13.
43 Skinner, 59–61.
44 De Cleene II:48–9, citing De Gubernatis, 35–8.
45 Rich, 60.
46 De Cleene, I:131.
47 Daniels and Stevans, II:809.
48 Friend, 299–300.
49 De Cleene, I:131.
50 Ibid.
51 Folkard, 106.
52 Ibid.
53 De Cleene, I:131, citing *Verband Deutscher Verain*, 1,350.
54 Baker, *Folklore of Plants*, 25.
55 Tongue, 27.
56 De Cleene, I:143.
57 Betony in North America refers to the genus Pedicularis, but in Britain and Europe to genus Stachys.
58 Lecouteux, 194.
59 Bonser, 350–63. Lecouteux, 194.
60 Grieve, I:97. Lecouteux, 194, citing a fourteenth-century Greek text, Hildegard of Bingen, and Platearius.
61 Gauntlet, 283. Rankine points out that this spell appears later in Lady Ayscough's *Book of Receipts and Chirurgery* (1692), later reproduced by Charles Dickens in *Household Words V* (1852).
62 Bonser, 350–63.
63 De Cleene, I:154–5.
64 De Cleene, I:154.
65 Becker et al., 113.
66 Landsell, 149.
67 Barber, 37–9. Also *The Khazar*.
68 Ryan, 198.
69 Bane, 30.
70 Tongue, 31.
71 Hatfield, 32.
72 Davies, 153.
73 McCleery et al. [online].
74 De Cleene, I:168–70.
75 Grieve, I:125.
76 Hatfield, 58.
77 Chapman, II:437, citing Turner.
78 Vickery, *Dictionary*, 393–4.
79 Skinner, 270.

80 Vickery, *Dictionary*, 60, citing Le Sueur, 91.

81 Venus in early Culpeper editions.

82 Baker, *Folklore of Plants*, 38.

83 De Cleene II:167.

84 Picton, 'Chamomile'.

85 De Cleene, II:167.

86 Baker, *Folklore of Plants*, 40. Also Friend, 218.

87 Picton, 'Chamomile.' Also Friend, 343, 618.

88 Folkard, 106.

89 Daniels and Stevans, II:763.

90 Böhnert and Hahn, 930.

91 Gerard, 'Chaste Tree'.

92 Gauntlet, 299.

93 Brand, III:298, citing Butler, *Dry Dinner*.

94 Baker, *Folklore of Plants*, 41–2.

95 Vickery, *Dictionary*, 72.

96 Albertus, 21

97 Daniels and Stevans, II:777.

98 The true four-leaved clover is not to be confused with oxalis, the plant usually sold commercially as four-leafed clover.

99 Vickery, *Dictionary*, 71.

100 Vickery, *Dictionary*, 71, citing Melton (1620)

101 Dyer, 85.

102 Vickery, *Dictionary*, 72–3. Folkard, 288.

103 Vickery, *Dictionary*, 73.

104 Ibid.

105 Vickery, *Dictionary*, 73.

106 De Cleene, II:179.

107 De Cleene, II:176.

108 Folkard, 110. Dyer, 102.

109 De Cleene, II:176.

110 Baker, *Folklore of Plants*, 43.

111 Dyer, 98.

112 Reade, 106-7.

113 Friend, 46.

114 Baker, *Folklore of Plants*, 102, with the rhyme given in full.

115 MacLeod, 24.

116 Tongue, 33.

117 Rich, 124.

118 Folkard, 101. Watts, 336, with references.

119 Daniels and Stevans, II:779. De Cleene, II:511.

120 Folkard, 108.

121 Stevans, II:779. Baker, *Folklore of Plants*, 47.

122 Folkard, 103.

123 De Cleene, I:401.

124 Baker, *Folklore of Plants*, 47.

125 De Cleene, I:403.

126 De Cleene, I:403, citing Teirlinck.

127 De Cleene, I:403.

128 Daniels and Stevans, II:779.

129 Albertus, 18.

130 Ibid.

131 Tongue, 33. Hatfield, 93.

132 Tongue, 33, citing 'a maid from Bruton, 1907'.

133 Rich, 140.

134 Folkard, 104. Against witchcraft, Daniels and Stevans, II:781. Also Rich, 140–41.

135 Daniels and Stevans, II:781. Davies, 155.

136 Daniels and Stevans, II:781.

137 Folkard 92. For Somerset, see Tongue, 30–31.

138 Gauntlet, 289.

139 Friend, 39.

140 Skinner, 105–6.

141 Ibid.

142 Friend, 40.

143 Baker, *Rural England*, 67.

144 Folkard, 103. Scotland: Brand III, 284, citing a seventeenth-century translation of *Anatomy of the Elder*.

145 Baker, *Folklore of Plants*, 55.

146 All information here is from De Cleene, I:244–5. Latter points also made in Baker, *Folklore of Plants*, 162.

147 Rich, 142. De Cleene, II:227. For Somerset, Baker, *Folklore of Plants*, 57.

148 De Cleene, II:227.

149 Friend, 362.

150 Friend, 361.

151 Dyer, 89.

152 Skinner, 110.

153 Brand, I:314–15.

154 Friend, 281–2, citing Dean
　　Jackson.
155 Skinner, 110.
156 Daniels and Stevans, II:785.
157 Skinner, 112–13.
158 Northcote, 177.
159 De Cleene, I:257.
160 Skinner, 112–13.
161 Culpeper editions vary.
162 Skinner, 113.
163 Skinner, 114–15.
164 Skinner, 114.
165 Ibid.
166 Tongue 33, citing Willett.
167 Lecouteux, 240–41.
168 Davies, 156.
169 Daniels and Stevans II: 'Garlic'.
170 Tongue, 162. Baker, *Folklore of
　　Plants*, 145.
171 Hatfield, 161.
172 Vickery, *Garlands*, 51.
173 Davies, 37.
174 Tongue, 162. Other examples in
　　Baker, *Folklore of Plants*, 68–71.
175 Friend, 186.
176 Tongue, 162.
177 De Cleene, I:298.
178 Friend, 286–7.
179 Skinner, 134.
180 Percy, III:263.
181 Skinner, 132.
182 Baker, *Folklore of Plants*, 73.
183 Folkard, 103.
184 Brand, III:333.
185 Davies, 43. De Cleene, I:311.
186 Dyer, 61.
187 Baker, *Folklore of Plants*, 75.
188 Gordon, 100.
189 De Cleene, II:260.
190 Ibid.
191 Ibid.
192 Baker, *Folklore of Plants*, 75.
193 Albertus, 21
194 De Cleene, II:261.
195 Lawton, 103. Dietz, 395. Baker,
　　75–6.
196 Tongue, 32. Baker, *Folklore of
　　Plants*, 75.
197 Anon., 'Herb Paris', *Metropolitan
　　Museum Blog*.
198 Grigson, Herb paris.
199 Tongue, 34, citing Roebuck,
　　'Quantock Hills'.
200 De Cleene, I:332–5.
201 De Cleene, I:335.
202 Baker, *Folklore of Plants*, 78.
203 Watt, 194. Baker, *Folklore of
　　Plants*, 78.
204 Tongue, 28. De Cleene, I:333–4.
205 Friend, 271. Also Folkard, 379.
206 Friend, 534.
207 Friend, 272.
208 Dyer, 77.
209 Brand, III:314.
210 Northcote, 178.
211 De Gurbernatis, 174. Northcote,
　　178. De Cleene, I:274.
212 De Cleene, I:354–5.
213 Tongue, 28. De Cleene, I:353.
　　Baker, *Folklore of Plants*, 83.
214 De Cleene, I:354.
215 De Cleene I:354, citing De
　　Gubernatis, 195–8, and Teirlinck,
　　327.
216 De Cleene, I:351.
217 Friend, 105. Folkard, 395–7.
　　Palmer, *Somerset*, 62, for West
　　Country.
218 Folkard, 395.
219 De Cleene, I:365.
220 Baker, *Folklore of Plants*, 85–6.
　　Whitlock, 110.
221 Brand I:13; III:274. Watts, 215.
222 Baker, *Folklore of Plants*, 85–6.
223 Folkard, 396. Watts, 215.
224 Baker, *Folklore of Plants*, 85–6.
225 Skinner, 145.
226 Skinner, 145. Folkard, 395.
227 Skinner, 145. Folkard, 395.
228 Daniels and Stevans, II:808.
　　Attribution to Highlands is from
　　Mac Coitir, 280.
229 Culpeper editions vary.
230 De Cleene, I:387.
231 Knab, 139.
232 Daniels and Stevans, II:812.
233 Skinner, 157–8.
234 Skinner, 159–60.
235 Rich, 11.

236 Friend, 292–5, 532–3. Dyer, 64–5, who quotes Lord Bacon and Coles, *Art of Simpling*, as well as Ben Jonson *Masque of Queens*.

237 Folkard, 108.

238 De Cleene, II:361.

239 Baker, *Folklore of Plants*, 96.

240 De Cleene, II:361.

241 Folkard, 433.

242 Skinner, 176.

243 Venus in early Culpeper editions.

244 Friend, 149–50.

245 Skinner, 178–9.

246 Rich, 22.

247 Rich, 27.

248 De Cleene, II:368.

249 De Cleene, I:415. Friend, 74–5.

250 Brand, III:16, quoting Coles, *Art of Simpling*.

251 Skinner, 179–81.

252 Baker, *Folklore of Plants*, 100.

253 Ibid.

254 Lecouteux, 196–7.

255 De Cleene, II:390.

256 Tongue, 33.

257 Folkard, 173.

258 Rich, 21.

259 De Cleene, II:391.

260 Northcote, 182. Tongue, 33.

261 Grieve, II:556.

262 Ibid.

263 Ibid.

264 Lecouteux, 192.

265 Lecouteux, 196–7.

266 Skinner, 190–91.

267 Tongue, 33.

268 Friend, 16.

269 De Cleene, I:467–9.

270 Skinner, 195–6. Folkard, 170.

271 Skinner, 197.

272 Dyer, 86.

273 Tongue, 166.

274 Culpeper did translate a book which gave olive trees to Jupiter on account of their jovial nature: *The Idea of Practical Physick* (1657). 1826 Gleave edn gives it to the Sun; Sibly and an 1807 edn give it to Venus.

275 Skinner, 202–3. De Cleene, I:506.

276 Culpeper says it is cold and moist, and useful for venereal complaints. Hence, lunar.

277 Rich, 10–11.

278 All from De Cleene, II:86.

279 Lecouteux, 107.

280 Lecouteux, 236.

281 Brand, III:314, citing Coles, *The Art of Simpling*, 68.

282 Skinner, 215–16. Baker, *Folklore of Plants*, 117.

283 Folkard, 108.

284 Northcote, 111.

285 Baker, *Folklore of Plants*, 121.

286 De Cleene, II:468.

287 Ibid.

288 De Cleene, II:468.

289 De Cleene, II:469.

290 De Cleene, II:468.

291 Ibid., II:468.

292 Folkard, 105. For Lancashire, Harland and Wilkinson, 71–2.

293 Rich, 141. Quoted in full in Harland and Wilkinson, 71, who attribute it to a manuscript preserved in Chetham's Library in Manchester, and which includes the instruction about fifteen days.

294 Baker, *Folklore of Plants*, 121. Watts, 348.

295 Culpeper editions vary in how they attribute Pine: some say Mars, some Sun. Lilly gives pine to Jupiter, but then later gives the pine tree itself to Saturn. The Saturn rulership is from two things: the pine is sacred to Dionysos, a goat god, the astral goat is Capricorn, ruled by Saturn. Moreover, Saturn rules dark and desolate places such as pine woods.

296 De Cleene, I:552.

297 Skinner, 217–18.

298 Skinner, 218.

299 Skinner, 217.

300 Culpeper editions vary.

301 Gauntlet, 299.

302 Skinner, 224–5.

303 Gauntlet, 299.
304 Folkard, 108.
305 Tongue, 33.
306 De Cleene, II:501.
307 Tongue, 33, citing Willett.
308 Tongue, 162. Baker, *Folklore of Plants*, 126.
309 De Cleene, II:501.
310 Folkard, 508. Grieve, II:660. Brand, III:300.
311 Folkard, 108.
312 Friend, 37.
313 Skinner, 231.
314 Greek origin story: Rich, 120–21. Roman origin story: Rich, 120–121. History of the rose in lore and symbolism: Rich, 171–6. Sacredness to Venus, and to silence: Friend, 212–14. Many rose stories: Skinner, 232–60.
315 Baker, *Folklore of Plants*, 129–32.
316 Rich, 53–4.
317 Tongue, 166.
318 De Cleene, I:626
319 Northcote, 129–30.
320 Friend, 217.
321 Baker, *Folklore of Plants*, 132–3. Vickery, *Dictionary*, 318–19. Briggs, 119.
322 De Cleene, I:645.
323 Dyer, 97.
324 De Cleene I:648
325 Baker, *Folklore of Plants*, 132–3.
326 Skinner, 260–61.
327 Baker, *Folklore of Plants*, 132–3. Brand, III:282.
328 Friend, 284.
329 De Cleene, I:659.
330 Friend, 273.
331 Dyer, 67, citing the ballad which appeared in 'Northumberland Garland'.
332 Dyer, 68.
333 De Cleene, I:660–61.
334 Thompson, 113. Howells, 178.
335 Vickery, *Garlands*, 58, 63. De Cleene, I:660–61.
336 Folkard, 103. Palmer, 62. Tongue, 28. Specifics of time of year, see Harland and Wilkinson, 72.
337 Friend, 284. Vickery, *Dictionary*, 321. Tongue, 166.
338 Thompson, 113. Howells, 178.
339 Friend, 534.
340 Sage was considered a plant of Jupiter in ancient times: De Cleene II:666. Rich, 115.
341 Briggs, 119.
342 De Cleene, II:668.
343 Dyer, 63. Thompson, 97.
344 Skinner, 265–6.
345 Hatfield, 315.
346 Folkard, 112.
347 Folkard, 104.
348 Friend, 274–5.
349 Folkard, 103.
350 Ibid.
351 Friend, 147. Brand, I:307.
352 De Cleene, II:445.
353 Skinner, 264.
354 De Cleene, II:445.
355 Baker, *Folklore of Plants*, 141.
356 De Cleene, II:445, translation rendered into modern English.
357 De Cleene, II:457.
358 Friend, 150.
359 Lecouteux, 107.
360 De Cleene, I:697.
361 Folkard, 566.
362 De Cleene, I:699.
363 De Cleene, I:697–9.
364 De Cleene, I:697. Baker, 149–50.
365 Gauntlet, 300–302.
366 Folkard, 109.
367 Folkard, 108. Baker, *Folklore of Plants*, 152.
368 Baker, *Folklore of Plants*, 152.
369 Gauntlet, 302. A very similar spell is on 303.
370 De Cleene, II:530.
371 De Cleene, II:531.
372 De Cleene, II:530.
373 Dyer, 55–6.
374 Albertus, 23.
375 Lecouteux, 107, citing Pseudo-Apuleius, *Herbarium*, which says the verbena must be collected during the waning moon and when the moon is in the first decan of Taurus or Scorpio.

376 De Cleene, II:530–31.
377 Folkard, 574.
378 Lecouteux, 222.
379 De Cleene, II:530–31.
380 De Cleene, II:530. Baker, *Folklore of Plants*, 153.
381 Hatfield, 355, citing an Elizabethan MS in Chetham's Library, Manchester.
382 De Cleene, II:532.
383 Friend, 610.
384 Albertus, 23.
385 Folkard, 574.
386 Ovid, *Fasti*. Ovid's source text, Livy's *The History of Rome* (I:24 and XXX:34), makes it clear that in war it is used for the ambassador's crown—the person who could safely enter enemy territory to negotiate or finalise treaties. Frazer, II:160.
387 Albertus, 23.
388 Ibid.
389 Baker, *Folklore of Plants*, 153.
390 Skinner, 290.
391 De Cleene, I:711. Baker, *Folklore of Plants*, 156.
392 Folkard, 582–5.
393 Quote is from Skinner, 290.
394 Tongue, 28.
395 Folkard, 584.
396 Skinner, 290.
397 Ibid.
398 Daniels and Stevans, II:862.
399 Daniels and Stevans, II:863.
400 Folkard, 586–7.
401 Brand I:105, quoting Thomas Fuller, *Worthies* (Cambridgeshire), 144.
402 Daniels and Stevans, 862.
403 De Cleene, I:731.
404 Daniels and Stevans, 863.
405 De Cleene, I:731.
406 Simpson, 59.
407 Modern herbal magician Scott Cunningham gave it to Mars, which I would not follow.
408 De Cleene, II:557, translation modernised.
409 All information in this entry is from II:557.
410 Tongue, 32. Also Daniels and Stevans, II:863, without regional attribution.
411 Hatfield, 382.
412 Baker, *Folklore of Plants*, 18.
413 Vickery, *Dictionary*, 406–8. Also Folkard, 588–9.
414 Baker, *Folklore of Plants*, 8, quoting Halliwell's *Popular Rhymes*. More dreaming spells: Vickery, *Dictionary*, 406–8. Folkard, 588–9 has two similar spells with words.
415 Daniels and Stevans, II:863.
416 Thompson, 97.
417 From the Hebrides. Baker, *Folklore of Plants*, 8–9.
418 Folkard, 588–9.
419 Vickery, *Dictionary*, 406–8.
420 Northcote, 180.
421 Baker, *Folklore of Plants*, 8–9.
422 Baker, *Folklore of Plants*, 163.
423 De Cleene, I:745–6.
424 De Cleene, I:746. Baker, *Folklore of Plants*, 163.
425 Skinner, 261–2. Folkard, 104.
426 Dyer, 69–70, citing Black, *Folk Medicine*, 202.
427 Skinner, 261–2.
428 Baker, *Folklore of Plants*, 149–50.
429 Northcote, 178, citing De Gubernatis, who in turn is citing a text dated c.1750.
430 Baker, *Folklore of Plants*, 96.
431 Albertus, 6.
432 Albertus, 8.
433 Rich, 168.
434 Albertus, 4.
435 Baker, *Folklore of Plants*, 149.
436 Folkard, 101–2.
437 Albertus, 13.
438 Albertus, 4–5.
439 Albertus, 16.
440 Gauntlet, 254.
441 Gauntlet, 288–9.

About the Author

CHRISTINA OAKLEY HARRINGTON is the founder of Treadwell's Books in London. A former academic historian, she now manages the shop's lecture series and special projects. Her interest in folk magic dates back to her childhood. In addition to *The Treadwell's Book of Plant Magic,* Harrington is the author of *Dreams of Witches.*

To Our Readers

Weiser Books, an imprint of Red Wheel/Weiser, publishes books across the entire spectrum of occult, esoteric, speculative, and New Age subjects. Our mission is to publish quality books that will make a difference in people's lives without advocating any one particular path or field of study. We value the integrity, originality, and depth of knowledge of our authors.

Our readers are our most important resource, and we appreciate your input, suggestions, and ideas about what you would like to see published.

Visit our website at www.redwheelweiser.com, where you can learn about our upcoming books and free downloads, and also find links to sign up for our newsletter and exclusive offers.

You can also contact us at info@rwwbooks.com or at

Red Wheel/Weiser, LLC
65 Parker Street, Suite 7
Newburyport, MA 01950

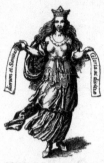

Treadwell's

✿   Treadwell's—often called "the most famous occult bookshop in the world"—is both a bookstore and events space located in the heart of London's historical Bloomsbury neighborhood, right behind the British Museum. Founded by Christina Oakley Harrington in 2003, Treadwell's quickly developed a packed schedule of scholarly lectures, practical magic classes, and late-night parties. Its legendary shopfloor is a salon of dark wood book cases and upholstered sofas, with a replica mummy case standing in the corner. The downstairs events space features William Morris inspired wallpapered walls and the fireplace of the Edwardian occultist Pamela Colman Smith, an artist who achieved fame for her painting of the Rider-Waite tarot deck. Workshops and courses are now offered on site and online, taught by longstanding practitioners and respected researchers.

✿   The shop's book selection is curated by the knowledgeable staff, to ensure it always offers the best publications on esoteric subjects. The Rare Books department offers a range of printed treasures and quirky secondhand titles, in an ever-changing selection. *The Treadwell's Book of Plant Magic* is the shop's first publication.

✿   Treadwell's founder Christina Oakley Harrington remains a guiding light and active presence aided by a bright, friendly, hardworking team of subject experts. To learn more visit Treadwell's at *www.treadwells-london.com*